Health and Weight Loss Companion

Valerie H. Lunden, M.A.

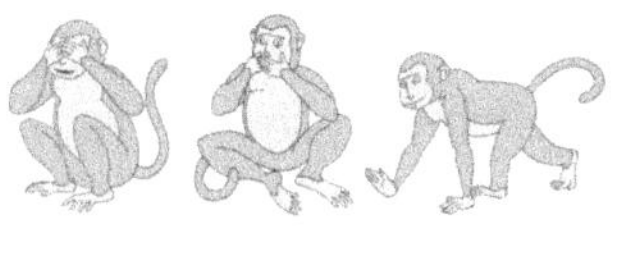

Monkey Mentors™

Health and Weight Loss Companion

www.brightperformance.com

Book design: Jim Bisakowski www.bookdesign.ca

Library of Congress Cataloging-in-Publication Data available upon request.

Lunden, Valerie H.

Bright Performance Ltd.

ISBN - 978-0-9822539-0-8

Published in the United States of America

Disclaimer

Readers are advised to consult with their physician or other medical practitioner before implementing the suggestions that follow. The information contained in this book is not intended as medical advice.

The authors, publishers, and/or distributors will not assume responsibility for any adverse consequences or liability resulting from any health or lifestyle changes described herein.

Dedication

To dearest Joy,
my friend, my muse, and my guiding light.

Contents

Monkey Do

"In fact, at the heart of the new consciousness lies the transcendence of thought, a newfound ability of rising above thought, of realizing a dimension within yourself that is infinitely more vast than thought. You then no longer derive your identity, your sense of who you are, from the incessant stream of thinking that in the old consciousness you take to be yourself."

—Eckhart Tolle
A New Earth

Introduction

A Love Story

I came from humble beginnings. My parents were not affluent, but we always ate well and food of any kind established how we gathered together and socialized with our friends. As a result of my love for food, during my youth I gained weight.

My family had immigrated to England when I was five years old. Moving from the East to the West, I was introduced to many new experiences, which included a host of brand-new culinary delights.

It was only in my adulthood that I realized that my personal food issues were not about scarcity but about abundance. Gaining weight had more to do with my taste for certain foods combined with the emotional impact of certain distinct events.

I remember always having open access to every sweet imaginable. Also, my young and eager mind was more than willing to try everything, particularly all the different varieties of candy.

There is one particular food memory that stands out above the rest during those early years and well into my teens. Every day before my father came home from work, he would stop at one of the shops at the local train station and buy a bar of chocolate. England was famous for the brand Cadbury. There was a large selection, and most of the bars were wrapped in shiny foil and divided into neat squares.

There wasn't a single evening that passed when my father didn't come home with one of those Cadbury bars stuffed deep down in his coat pocket. Of course, this bar was supposed to be shared with the rest of the family, but I believed (and still do) that he had bought that chocolate bar just for me. I also believed that this was his way of expressing his love.

When I would see him turn the corner of our street, I would rush to meet him, and with eagerness, I would search through his coat until I unearthed my treat. This was our ritual, a ritual that ended with him laughing out loud and then kissing me on the cheek.

After dinner, the family would each get his or her square of chocolate, and I would get what was left over. Being a dutiful child, I was put in charge of divvying up the portions. To be honest, this chore was unpleasant because I really didn't want to share.

This chocolate gift came to mean more than just rituals remembered. After decades of being overweight, I finally understood how the taste of chocolate represented love, or more precisely, the removal of love from my life. Like a few other cherished foods, chocolate symbolized something lost, the loss of my father's love after he died.

I remember those times, years later, when I literally gorged on chocolate, not even appreciating the flavor. After eating my fill, nothing much had changed except the excess amount of calories I had consumed.

Soon after my father died, I began to eat large quantities of sweets; sometimes I couldn't stop and would become ill. Each sweet taste became a source of instant love. My mind had somehow bound together an emotion with a memory and interpreted this connection as the need for a specific food.

Sometime during my adulthood, the connection between chocolate and love changed. Eating chocolate no longer represented happy times and familiar rituals but assuaging a certain form of unhappiness, a reversal in meaning of the original emotional connection, which was love.

While keeping a daily thought log, I noticed other food patterns emerging, particularly during unhappy moments when I gravitated to certain "special" foods. Writing about these thoughts uncovered deeper emotions and food triggers, and exposed the underlying causes for my weight gain.

Incorporating a series of non-food-related practices produced positive eating behaviors. Over time, chocolate no longer became associated with shiny foil wrappers, a comforting taste, or the sound of familiar male laughter. A new clarity arrived, and this grew stronger as I paid more attention to what I was feeling. With continued focus, the connection between taste and unhappy memories became stronger, and overeating became less frequent.

Today, chocolate remains a delicious treat, but no longer a living reminder of a moment in time that has come and gone.

~ ~ ~

Monkey See

Chapter One

Creating Visual Focus

Who Are the Weight Loss Monkeys?

The ability to mimic human behaviors extends to a few creatures in the animal world. The most well known of these are apes and monkeys. For example, chimpanzees, who are "great apes" share 98.76 percent gene similarity to humans in their DNA.[1] They are able to mimic, repeat and imitate humans, an example of this being their ability to learn and communicate using American Sign Language.

The three fictional Weight Loss Monkeys that embody the health initiative in this book are called See, Say, and Do. They each represent certain healing tools that complement the sensory relationships that we have with negative food behaviors.

During my personal health initiative, I was able to improve my weight loss by becoming aware of my emotional, negative reactions to food. These thoughts were connected to "special" foods that when eaten initiated overeating.

By observing my relationships to these "special" foods, I was able to isolate key feelings and behaviors that triggered negative responses and affected the success of my diets.

In contrast, wild monkeys do not experience broad-spectrum feelings. Their sense of awareness is primitive compared to ours. It is based on keen instincts and a honed sense of survival, expressed through repetitive behaviors. Examples of this include eating the same foods and not venturing far from their natural habitat unless forced to do so by environmental impacts.

This book, as well as the entire Monkey series, embraces one premise: identifying those repetitive behaviors that disrupt our goals, particularly when it comes to weight loss and better health. These eating behaviors are formed because of emotional food events, which resurface as powerful memories created in our past.

I should mention that the Weight Loss Monkeys each represent both the best and worst of these repetitive behaviors. In my experience, it was the consistent practice of both the best and the worst that caused me to stop dieting and return to age-old eating habits. By identifying these food relationships, I was able to limit the distractions that affected my diet routine.

The Best Way to Use This Book

I developed the Health and Weight Loss Companion for individuals like myself who struggle with weight loss and are unable to maintain stable health goals. The process within this book encourages writing and other sensory tools, which can be used to improve the results of almost any commercial diet or health initiative.

Make it a practice to write notes in this book. If you require permission to do so, you have it. There are no guidelines for these personal notes unless you create them yourself. For those of you who beg for order in your lives, the only suggestion is to write as neatly as possible, because you may need to review these notes on a regular basis. If you require extra space, blank pages have been added at the end of each chapter.

Every one of your notes is important. Positive food thoughts make sense, but also pay attention to those thoughts that take you off your diet and initiate emotional eating. From a weight loss perspective, what matters is having increased awareness and being able to identify when changes are necessary to improve the results of your plan.

As I continued to use the Monkey tools, my focus improved. After identifying the emotion and taste triggers that produced cravings, I was able to recognize how often any single combination of memory and taste would cause me to cheat on my diet. Another productive outcome was being able to reread my notes and remind myself which thoughts to focus on every day. This included all of those positive experiences that I often forgot to appreciate, such as the actual weight I had lost.

Finally, I experienced the gift of time. I was no longer impatient to get to the weight loss finish line, and I had sufficient awareness to follow a customized health plan.

Why the See Monkey Is Important

Awareness for most of us begins with the visual, how we see ourselves as we fit into our clothes and our world. There were times in my life when I forgot that I was overweight, and this caused me to gain even more weight and compromise my health.

I remember buying clothes that fit me no matter what shape I carried. I would look in the mirror and see my body, the body that I was used to seeing. What I never saw was the thin me, because I had never appreciated my body image.

The scale was another visual tool. When I weighed myself, I could see only the numbers on the scale. My mind could not focus on the numbers that made the difference, the numbers that represented a lighter me.

From movies, pictures, and magazines, I understood that other people weighed less and wore smaller clothes sizes, but these ideals were nowhere close to my own confused reality.

After incorporating the Monkey tools described in this book, I slowly began to view my body and health with what felt like a new set of eyes. This perspective was not associated with some fantasy about my appearance but was focused on what I actually looked like.

I would read a few of my handwritten notes every night before going to bed and even before I sat down to eat meals.

Another way I used the companion was to choose my dining partners. By having more diet focus, I was able to select people and food experiences that supported healthier eating.

Building Monkey Momentum

The other two Weight Loss Monkeys, Say and Do, are responsible for establishing new diet behaviors using continuous motivation.

After I received the benefits of the writing tool, I added another tool and then another. Instead of being quiet and secretive about my process, I became more confident, and I was able to talk about my weight loss with my food mentors. I told them how I wanted to reach my health objectives and asked them for their encouragement and support.

I discovered that after my weight loss goals had been established and reinforced with positive thoughts, I could stay on my diet with fewer interruptions.

Combined with consistent action (making use of the tools), it became difficult, perhaps next to impossible, to neglect this new weight loss perspective. Taste no longer became heightened. I cheated less; I exercised more; and I became both accountable and resourceful when it came to food choices. Even the actual food management component became easier.

The repetitive lifestyle of yo-yo dieting became an afterthought. I no longer purchased diet books unless I was doing research for this book. The best part was that by having more positive focus I now believed that my goal was achievable.

~ ~ ~

Monkey Chapter Notes

Creating Visual Focus

Chapter Two

Tools for the Journey

Monkey Inventory

During all those years of dieting, the only real diet tools I had at my disposal were the scale and exercise. I remember a few diets that advocated writing a food diary and even keeping track of consumed calories. However, after a few weeks, this practice became difficult, particularly when I ate away from home.

The use of a food diary helps to identify daily food consumption but does not explore the precise thoughts that connect these foods with our fragile emotions. Using the Monkey tools, I soon discovered that I had failed each of my diets because I was unable to manage my thoughts.

A Self-portrait

I had been overweight since my preteens. Being unhealthy affected many aspects of my life, from social events to shopping excursions, as well as the ability to do vigorous exercise. The range of unhappy food-related feelings was unlimited.

As you may have guessed by now, this Monkey book is not concerned with typical diets or daily diet activities; this book has been designed as a thought and behavior support tool.

In the past, I had been on countless diets, and I had been unfocused on all of them. I never once identified with the thoughts that created my poor self-image. These same thoughts kept me from visualizing myself as a thin, healthy person.

The weight loss miracle that exists in this book is the ability to simply pay attention. This may sound easy, but you will soon discover that the power of food thoughts control how a chronic dieter lives his or her life.

After I started to connect taste with emotions, I also recorded how I chose my meals and when I neglected exercise.

Another surprise discovery was my perpetual interaction with food. I thought about food all the time, and I never forgot to eat, even when I wasn't hungry.

The Monkey Experience

So what does it mean to be healthy? Based on the diets written and advertised, there are so many variations on this theme.

As mentioned, the Weight Loss Monkeys' goal is to first create the best thought environment possible, one that promotes a focus on health.

In the wild monkeys are healthy, and they don't eat three meals a day. They also don't think about food the same way people do. In the book Green for Life[2] by Victoria Boutenko, she describes how chimpanzees are happiest eating green, leafy vegetables as well as fruits. They eat bananas, not just to satisfy a source of potassium, but as a nutritionally satisfying part of their overall diet.

In contrast, I thought about food a minimum of three times a day. I ate when I was full, and then if I felt like it, I would eat again! I believe that my food behaviors are very similar to many others who struggle with unresolved weight issues.

See Monkey Observations

With the advancement of television, computers, and the Internet, we have become a more visual planet. In the diet world, no one will believe that you are on a diet unless actual results are visible.

There are no accurate statistics recorded that tell us how many people start diets, succeed, or fail. Accurate statistics do not exist for how many diets people try, when they try them, or what results they have. For the most part, the act of dieting is also strictly personal, which may preclude the gathering of accurate data.

As mentioned, diet success may be based upon a specific visual perspective, which is satisfied only by the exact moment when others start to notice our weight loss, or when the scale registers a much lower number, or when we fit into clothes that are of a smaller size. One of the only non-visual criteria for diet success is when your doctor says you have reached your goal.

Interruption factors vary, but dieters also give up on diets because they don't see the results.

Monkey Tools: Diet Thoughts Log

Okay, what are you thinking right now?

Have you written it down? Could it be that you are regretting picking up this book? Is that the thought that will stop you from reading on?

Similar stop-thoughts arrive in our consciousness all the time. These stop-thoughts represent defense mechanisms derived by our brains to protect us from making mistakes. However, they can also stop us from moving forward and making progress.

A template for the thoughts log, Figure 1, is provided in this chapter. The Weight Loss Monkeys urge you to make copies of the template and record your food perceptions. It may surprise you just how often you think about food.

This tool tracks diet success and supports greater focus. Later in this book, the Weight Loss Monkeys will discuss daily weigh-ins and why these numbers should be added to your log.

As they happen, also add your thoughts about weight gain and weight loss to the thoughts log. What is written in the log is specific to your personal experiences and how food impacts various aspects of your life.

The template has a column labeled, Contributions. This column can be used to add positive food responses. It can also be used for thoughts that you might not readily acknowledge. An example might be: "I hate iceberg lettuce." An alternative thought might be: "Why do I hate iceberg lettuce? It really does taste good when I prepare it properly to create a delicious salad."

The thoughts log is used to create awareness and change food perceptions so that we can make healthier food decisions.

The Weight Loss Monkeys realize that in the beginning stages, having increased positive food thoughts may be challenging, but this practice, when continued, can improve understanding and reinforce reasons for healthier eating.

Monkey Questions: Observer

- Write one paragraph about how you feel about the thoughts log and why.
- Will it be a waste of your time to write about your food thoughts? Why do you think this? Is what you think really true?
- In the past, have you reached your health goals by believing these food thoughts?
- Write a detailed response about where you learned these food thoughts. This may require some in-depth memory searching.

Monkey Chapter Summary

Positive food thoughts develop over time. In the early stages of a traditional diet, it is usually enthusiasm that supports initial weight loss. After this phase, positive thinking and increased focus become critical to overcoming future weight gain and the tendency for most dieters to terminate their diets.

Most diets, when followed, can achieve weight loss. Most fat and calorie-reduction plans, when fully participated in, will not only drop pounds but also reduce inches and produce that all-important visual response that we are seeking from other people.

The thoughts log monitors food thoughts. These are the thoughts that cause the dieter to stay on or end his or her diet. With continued and frequent use of the thoughts log, food awareness improves, and this in turn stimulates increased weight loss.

~ ~ ~

Monkey Thoughts Log Instructions

(1) Date of thought: Valuable for tracking recurring food thoughts.

(2) The actual food or diet thought and any description.

(3) Positive or negative: was this food thought helpful to your health plan or not?

(4) How to change this food thought so it better contributes to your health goal.

(5) Origination: History of the thought. What situation caused you to first think this food thought?

(6) Recurring thought (yes or no): how often do you have these same food thoughts? When did you last have this thought?

(7) Are these thoughts really true? Why do you believe this thought is true?

Monkey Thoughts Log						
Date (1)	Food or Diet Thought (2)	(+) or (-) (3)	Contribution to Health (4)	Origination (Explain) (5)	Recurring (Yes or No) (6)	True or False (7)

Figure 1. Monkey Thoughts Log (Make Copies)

Monkey Chapter Notes

Chapter Three

Monkey Taste Test

Not the Real Thing

I began an initiative versus a new diet because I wanted to achieve better health. The food plan I chose had nothing to do with tasty foods and everything to do with improving nutrition.

A visit to the local grocery store confirmed this health perspective. As I walked down aisle after aisle, I took note of all the low-fat variations of my favorite foods. There was low-fat bread, low-fat pizza and low-fat butter. The complete list of these low-fat foods is too long to mention here, but if I wanted to eat a low-fat variation of any food it probably did exist.

Monkey Food

Food and diet industries have profited by simulating our favorite tastes in "healthier" versions. These tastes satisfy our emotional needs so that we continue to buy and eat food while supposedly achieving weight management.

These industries would like us to believe that having this food convenience is essential to both our happiness and social mobility. Instead, diet foods and foods created in low-fat, sugar-free, or other varieties are what the Weight Loss Monkeys consider both temporary solutions and health distractions. The main problem with recreated, fictional foods is that they continue to connect us to unhealthy food memories.

Several of the diet programs I used in the past allowed me to eat low-calorie meals. At the time, it was easy to embrace these diets because I could eat just like everybody else and not feel deprived.

In reality, this was the actual problem. I continued the same eating behaviors, learning nothing in terms of what my body needed for improved nutrition.

It is partly because of these fictional foods that our health perspective has become disconnected from the nutritional needs of our bodies, which has resulted in an overweight and unhealthy global society.

In my situation, fictional foods would always be inferior to the actual foods they were substituting. Another complex issue was that certain food tastes, no matter how they were presented, caused me to overeat. For example, chocolate had a direct connection to my need to find a source of love. As you will read later in this chapter, pizza had a strong emotional connection to friendship.

Continuing to eat even those "healthier" versions did nothing more than confirm that my unconscious food states would return and I would resume unhealthy eating habits.

Valuing Friendship

Food dates have been ongoing in my life since I moved away from home in the early eighties. I describe these sessions as having two components. The first was eating by myself; the second was eating certain foods while at home and alone.

Entries in my thoughts log uncovered eating habits that began as early as my teens. One of these food habits was eating meals in my bedroom, even when my family was at home. These private food experiences changed when I became an adult. At certain difficult moments in my life, I would make food dates with myself and eat certain foods associated with specific emotions.

These food dates occurred mostly when I was alone; however, when I craved something that I could not prepare myself, I would dine out.

My last formal overeating experience resulted in writing this chapter. This happened during another high-emotion period in my life. I had had a major disagreement with one of my good friends. We had not talked for several weeks, and I was feeling a great deal of guilt and unhappiness.

The overeating behaviors began to surface when my unhappy emotions had reached a peak. I made the decision to go grocery shopping. This in itself was not an unusual event; however, during this particular shopping excursion, I purchased only decadent and high-calorie foods that I never ate by myself.

The following day, I made another unconscious decision to stay at home, a form of solitary confinement. In the space of four hours, I watched several movies and ate two medium-sized pizzas. This was immediately followed by eating two decadent desserts.

After consuming all of this food, I immediately became tired and went to bed, four hours before my usual bedtime.

In contrast, the following day seemed almost surreal. It was business as usual. I woke up early and exercised. I ate according to my health initiative and remained on program for the next two weeks without cheating.

It was shocking to realize that my thoughts had combined to form a cohesive plan. Like foot soldiers preparing to go to war, my food thoughts had somehow organized, ready to do battle with the sadness and pain I had stored away.

Pizza had always been a favorite food; however, I never realized that the look and taste of pizza was associated with friendship. When I missed my friends, I ate pizza. I seldom ate pizza alone, and I had never eaten two pizzas in one sitting.

My emotions had resulted in an outpouring of grief. As I ate those pizzas, I felt less lonely, and during those four hours of overeating, I temporarily stopped suffering the loss of my dear friend.

I only became conscious of this event two weeks after my emotions had stabilized and I had resumed my health initiative. This awareness came into being because I created and answered the questions included in this chapter.

I was already aware of how taste issues had deep and guarded associations with various emotions. This pizza experience not only taught me how organized my food thoughts were, but also confirmed that food tastes were interwoven with my memories. When these memories sprang to life, they did nothing more than put me into exile, eating all of those foods that had never supported my physical or emotional well-being.

Monkey Questions: Taste

- List all of your "special" foods.
- How often do you eat these "special" foods?
- How often have you eaten these foods during the last year?
- Explain why these foods are your favorites.
- As you eat these foods, what do you feel and why?
- Are these foods connected to any events, emotions, or people?
- When was the last time you ate these "special" foods with other people?
- Are there any foods that you eat when you are alone or when you think no one is watching?

Monkey Chapter Summary

The sensation of taste contributes to diet failure by keeping the dieter connected to certain food memories.

Improving food nutrition, losing weight, and leading a healthy lifestyle has little connection to the actual taste of food.

The biology of the body cannot differentiate between a hamburger and a salad, it is the mind that makes these distinctions. The body is only focused on the quality of food it is given, and reproduces these foods into carbohydrates, proteins, fats and sugars.

The diet industry produces low calorie/low fat food alternatives, which are not necessarily healthy alternatives because most of these foods are made with preservatives and other chemicals.

~ ~ ~

Monkey Chapter Notes

Chapter Four

Why Not Diet?

Did I Want to Lose Weight?

Diet was that four-letter word that made me feel anxious. When I was off the diet, I felt happy. That was until I found out that I had gained weight.

Beginning another diet guaranteed only one thing, that I would again have to give up all of my favorite foods. As the years passed and I gained more weight, the word again created feelings of lack that became the most uncomfortable aspect of starting any new health regimen.

How would I again live without bread, potatoes, chocolate, ice cream, and beef? Would I again have to eat more lettuce, drink "power" shakes, and in general eat less food?

Also, at some point, all of those usual and customary diet behaviors would again cause me to eat more unauthorized bars of chocolate (to numb my unhappiness).

This diet chatter had had free access to my thoughts for decades. The conversations would arrive when I became overwhelmed and unconscious, and the feelings that resulted would accompany me during weight gain and obesity.

There were other conversations that were equally influential and went something like this: "Why not take the weekend off? You can start the diet again on Monday." Another familiar conversation had two parts: "Just one extra slice of bread won't hurt. Why not a few bites of dessert as well?"

It wasn't like I'd never eaten dessert before or tasted the same dessert many times. I now had to ask myself, what was it that made me want to eat the same dessert over and over again?

I don't remember ever wanting extra servings of fruits or vegetables. In fact, the most restricted foods proved to be the most comforting and, of course, the easiest way to sabotage my diet.

From age thirteen to my mid-forties, these conversations continued. The result was that I never stuck to any plan long enough for it to work.

Even when it came to the actual diet practice, I became focused on that combination of taste and emotion, which entwined together, repeated as thoughts, and resulted in a chain of unhealthy eating behaviors.

The Joy of Living

My negative weight loss thoughts shifted to a positive health perspective during the summer of 2007. That year, I vacationed with one of my dear friends.

Spending time with her for several days allowed me to gain an entirely different perspective on why I ate food.

As long as I had known her, my friend had been disciplined about her health routine. This was in complete contrast to my own undisciplined food behaviors.

My friend was mostly a raw eater. She ate fruits and vegetables, avoided meat and dairy, and always made the healthiest food choices possible. At some point during our friendship, I had unconsciously labeled her as rigid when it came to the subject of food. I also believed that her overly zealous food behaviors would somehow ruin our vacation.

As it happened, all of my worrying was unnecessary, and this trip proved to be the most important food experience of my life.

Watching my friend's food behaviors made me understand the importance of nutrition. While she had been focused on overall health, I had been focused on body image and the numbers on a scale.

It was after this trip that I was placed in the unusual position of reviewing a lifetime of rules and biases about eating. I had no one to blame but myself for being overweight because I was the one who had made all of those bad food decisions. I had also created excuses for not exercising and to end diets when I believed they were not working. The most daunting realization was that I had started to negate my own self-worth because I was overweight.

After a month of focusing on my new health initiative, I lost weight, and the effort was not as difficult as I had imagined. During the next ten months, I lost twenty-five pounds. It was the most weight I had ever lost in my life, and this was the longest I had ever been on any plan.

I realized that during all of those decades of dieting and hating my body shape, it had been my thoughts that had always interrupted my weight loss. It had also been my thoughts that had caused me to focus on an external viewpoint, not a viewpoint that matched my innermost wants and desires.

Thoughts were just thoughts. Thoughts could be changed, particularly when they were creating unproductive health behaviors that were impacting how I lived my life.

Living the New Life

I remember how I used to criticize my friend's diet behaviors. In mixed company, I would often describe her as being overly compulsive. Quite rightly, she had ignored my remarks.

Even though I had been aware of her healthy attitude and subsequent food behaviors, I had ignored how committed she was to her diet practice. All of her food choices worked because they were combined in one flowing thought pattern. She may have had issues with food, but hers were completely different from mine.

She had always been slim and more comfortable with her body image than I had been. Most important, her food actions were never based on taste; they were focused on overall nourishment. During our vacation, I made it my objective to watch how she viewed her health. I concluded that all of the added fruits and vegetables, plus her dedication to exercise, were part of a stream of self-designed thoughts.

By habit, my friend also adapted to any dining experience while remaining vigilant (if not strict) about her health regimen. She was a true example of weight-management consciousness, even as her behaviors contradicted the behaviors of most dieters who never reach their goals.

Today, I describe my friend as thin, healthy, active, and social. She has friends aplenty and eats complete meals with all of them. Most important, during all of those fifteen years, she always fit into her clothes, and if that wasn't maddening enough, she has always worn the same size.

Another thing I could not quite get over was that she had never been on a formal diet. She (occasionally) ate bread, chocolate, and beef, and whenever offered anything decadent, she would enjoy every bite, even cleaning out her bowl of sorbet or gelato until the bowl looked virtually spotless!

My friend considered food a tool to be used to enhance her life. Food was not her companion, rival, confidant, or nemesis. Food never dictated what dress size she wore or what social engagement she attended. When it came to food and living a food-filled life, she did everything she wanted and went everywhere she wanted to go. She knew exactly what to order from the menu, and she relished each and every eating experience.

Even more significant, my friend was not plagued by ill health, weight issues, and social inadequacies about food. When it came to what she ate and how much she exercised, this had more to do with how her mind worked and how she focused her thoughts so that her body paid attention.

Monkey Weight Loss

The Weight Loss Monkeys are by nature inquisitive creatures, and being inquisitive is an important component of any diet.

In most cases, when we purchase diet books and begin diet programs, the inquisitive part of us has already envisioned a successful conclusion.

When I was dieting, I believed that each diet would work and that each diet would eliminate the misery of being overweight.

I often purchased diet books because they were recommended. I had noticed how other people had lost weight on these plans, and I wanted the same results.

As they are structured for consumers, most diets begin with instructions. My thoughts often had me flipping to the diet section first and ignoring the author's research and recipes. I believe this had more to do with my need to know what foods I would again be giving up before I committed to the plan.

As time would tell, such thoughts created limitations. I may have succeeded on any one of these plans if I had just read all of the instructions and stayed focused.

In each case, the diet merely represented a road map or tool. If used as designed, it may have helped me to reach my weight loss destination and to maintain a healthy weight.

Other People's Thoughts

Our diet rituals are also impacted by peer pressure. During my weight loss journey, peer pressure affected how I interacted with my slim friends. This influence extended to how I viewed celebrities, and led to feelings of envy toward people who had slim physiques and wore smaller clothes sizes. Because of a host of negative thoughts, I had formed unrealistic views about my own body image.

Most celebrities' appeal is intrinsic to how healthy and attractive they look both on screen and in public. Perhaps celebrities and certain famous people consider image and weight loss to be as important to their careers as many of us consider a college education to be important to getting a great job. However, the amount of effort taken to create this image is not always what the general public focuses on. Celebrities spend hours a day, every day, paying attention to how they look. How much time and attention are we willing to give to our diets and health plans? Understanding this question may help to identify the dieter's level of commitment to his or her own weight loss process.

The Cheating Monkey

During the early stages of my diets there would be faster weight loss, and my negative food thoughts would try to find ways to sabotage my progress. Losing weight meant that I could now afford to cheat, even just a little bit.

Over time, the cheating continued, and this particular pattern of behavior endured well beyond the diet. Cheating was the main reason why I lost focus, stopped the plan, and regained the weight.

The act of cheating encouraged cycles of behavior that only served to contradict my goal.

As it pertains to all of these diets, the lesson learned was that I had to stay on the plan, any plan that I enjoyed, and not give up.

Monkey Questions: Diet Choices

Do your best to write detailed responses to the following questions.

- List all of the diets and fads that you have heard about. Are they still popular today? If not, why not?
- Write one paragraph about your weight loss priorities. Rank these priorities in order of their importance.
- Which frequent thoughts have stopped you from completing your diets in the past?
- Which thoughts have caused you to regain the weight that you have lost?
- Is your objective to stay at a certain weight for the rest of your life? What is this weight goal, and why did you choose it?
- List every diet that you have tried and why you stopped each plan.
- How much time can you dedicate to your health every day? This includes time for food preparedness and exercise.

Monkey Chapter Summary

Certain foods, combined with the impact of strong emotions, are the primary catalysts that disrupt diet focus. The more focused the dieter's thoughts, the more permanent the weight loss.

A dieter's thoughts produce subtle influences (both positive and negative) that require strict attention.

Negative food thoughts can be formed during periods of intense emotion that cause an inability to manage the actual diet process.

Our modern Western society enjoys quick fixes, where permanence is contrary to change. Diets and diet fads are temporary measures that relieve weight loss anxiety but usually do not focus on improving nutrition.

Documenting diet thoughts encourages weight loss and improves overall health. Improving food focus includes paying close attention to the emotions that become stimulated by specific tastes.

The Weight Loss Monkeys advocate the use of focus tools such as the thoughts log, which helps to eliminate our dependency on quick-fix diets.

~ ~ ~

Monkey Chapter Notes

Chapter Five

Who Is Watching My Weight?

A Self-portrait

My friends usually don't mention anything when I gain weight; I suppose that is why they are my friends. First, it's not polite, and second, I suppose they don't want to hurt my feelings or risk our friendship.

The only time I can remember someone mentioning something negative about my body image was when I was thirteen and my mother told me that I should lose weight. Unfortunately, she never told me how.

My mother had always been a remote parent. When it came to outward expressions of affection, I wished we had a deeper relationship. Because I was always trying to please her, I decided to go on a diet. This would be the first of many, and I realize now that each of those diets had been focused on trying to get the attention of other people.

I remember once listening to a TV celebrity discussing her relationship with the grandmother who raised her. She described her grandmother as doing the best that she could based on what she knew at the time. After writing this book I realized that my mother had done her best to communicate to me how much she was worried about my health.

During that diet I lost five pounds in the first week. I was very excited and happy, but when I told my mother, she didn't offer any encouragement. I believe this was the initial moment when my thoughts connected with a negative food association.

There were no lessons learned during this diet experience except that I was physically unattractive to another person, an idea that became etched onto my soul.

Thirty years and many unsuccessful diets later, I came to the conclusion that I was the only person whose opinion mattered when it came to the acceptance of my body image. What others liked or disliked about me was of little importance to my health or my life. It also occurred to me that the past pain and negative thinking associated with my physical appearance were formed in the past and by other people's perceptions.

Moving Forward

Because I needed to understand my food thoughts, I came to the conclusion that any future diet had to embody a greater health consciousness.

There were several steps in this process, and none of them involved food. First, I created the Monkey tools, which stopped me from continuing the habit of yo-yo dieting. I also realized the body image I wanted wouldn't happen overnight, and any new weight lost would have to be permanent. For this to happen, I needed a reasonable food plan, and a way to stay on this plan no matter what thoughts I had.

In the Stands

In our Western society, there are many advocates for better health. Television, the media, pharmaceutical companies, and even diet programs all promote how easy it is to achieve the ideal body image. Unfortunately, millions of people still remain overweight, even with full access to all of this information. Indeed, weight loss, weight gain, and all the consequences that result have become burdens that now pose health risks.

For most of my life, I watched my weight as a spectator. The body image I had desired for decades was nothing more than a fictional representation of myself. My views were based on other people's perceptions, combined with the impact of various emotional events that had happened during my life.

With so many outside influences, sometimes I felt like everyone else was watching my weight except for me. In truth, other than my mother, no one was really watching my weight; I just thought they were.

Under these conditions, I had to ask myself, who did I think was watching my weight, and why did I think their opinions were important?

More Weight

Using my new tools, I discovered that being overweight was the result of a combination of certain life dynamics that had very little to do with overeating.

One of the Weight Loss Monkeys' perspectives is founded in the principle that thoughts impact overeating, which in itself is neither unusual nor a new phenomenon. The human ability to process billions of thoughts is also not a unique concept. However, when these mind processes are combined with emotion and taste triggers, weighing more cannot be blamed on just an abuse of food. Weighing more now has a close association with many other sensory experiences.

In contrast, as primitive creatures, wild monkeys do not have a wide variety of tasty foods to choose from, nor do they have complex emotions.

Compared to most people, their lives are simple, and their diets are equally simple. This diet consists of four main food categories, which are greens, fruits, blossoms, and insects.[2] Monkeys never worry about fat versus carbohydrates and proteins, or any other myriad of food combinations. In this regard, their food choices are focused on good nutrition, which can be described as a natural complement to their survival instinct.

As previously discussed, for people living in Western cultures, food consumption is also influenced by conditions such as stress, peer pressure, celebrity worship, joy, sadness, heritage, and daily lifestyle dynamics. These conditions create a multitude of thoughts that when combined with emotion result in excessive and unconscious eating, and is further complicated by the need to satisfy taste.

Health Issues

Perhaps the most pressing of concerns to the Weight Loss Monkeys is the decline in overall health. With age and environmental changes, the human body works less efficiently, and when it is being fed the wrong foods, overall health worsens.

The functioning of the human body becomes further jeopardized by excessive weight gain, which exerts pressure on the limbs, vital organs, and the skeleton, reducing the efficiency of normal body processes. Within the vast scope of these physical conditions, there is a heightened propensity for disease, as well as health conditions such as cancer and osteoporosis. This would seem contrary to living in an advanced scientific age; however, cures have not yet been discovered for these conditions.

Complicating this physiological dilemma, people tend to pay more attention to their day-to-day routines and neglect their health. The unfortunate reality is that there is not enough time to deal with everything, and taking care of our bodies is often last on the list of priorities.

Monkey Questions: The Watchers

- Make a list of all the people whom you believe affect your weight gain and weight loss.
- Why are these people so influential?
- Are these people movie stars, celebrities, family members, or some other group of individuals?
- What makes their opinions important to how you make your food decisions? Give examples.
- Are these people your age?

- How much time and effort do these people contribute to their own health?
- In your opinion, how do these people represent optimum health?
- If they do not represent optimum health, why do you consider these individuals important?
- Make a list of your food mentors. Are these the people who can encourage and support you during your weight loss journey?

Monkey Chapter Summary

A dieter's focus may become interrupted (or distracted) because of the thoughts and behaviors of other people, specifically people who have little or no say in the dieter's overall well-being.

The Weight Loss Monkeys' goal is to create a shift in focus, which allows the dieter to improve his or her overall thought environment. In this new thinking arena, negative food thoughts and thought distractions will have less influence. Much more significant, whoever was watching our weight in the past now becomes irrelevant.

Food in itself is uncomplicated, and the ability to provide the body with nutrition is equally uncomplicated.

Our emotional health is not in any way connected to food or nutrition, unless we allow our thoughts to make it so.

~ ~ ~

Monkey Chapter Notes

Chapter Six

Undirected Wants

A Self-portrait

Being overweight had impacted many aspects of my life. There are countless stories, including the times when people offered their unconscious, hurtful, and cruel remarks about my appearance. Once I had a male friend who told me he could not date me because he didn't like my body shape. There were other times when I felt disconnected from social experiences, not because of specific people, but because of the influence of a painful memory. All of these circumstances resulted in decades of eating far too much, far too often.

Overeating also produced many feelings of doubt and hopelessness. When these thoughts were at their most powerful, they resulted in long periods of self-isolation. Embarrassed with my body image, I often withdrew from society, staying home and eating comfort foods until I felt ill.

I describe these negative thought influences as undirected wants. They are memories that congregate as one or more powerful food expressions, which can recur, particularly in difficult emotional situations.

Undirected wants are unique to each person. My undirected wants connected me with the foods that were not part of my diet, and I ate these foods without consideration for my health or my body shape.

The primary reason why I was on a diet was to look better and regain my health. This became more difficult to accomplish when I continued to cling to negative food memories that had been created in my past.

Monkey Formation

One specific memory that became part of a negative congregation of thoughts had to do with my need to fit in with others. The incident goes back to my early twenties and a group of friends in California. These friends lived near the beach; the ocean was their back door. They were very good friends, and they often invited me to their house, which was a huge privilege.

At the time, going to the beach represented a recurring nightmare, particularly if I was required to wear minimal beach clothing such as swimsuits and shorts.

Every time my friends extended an invitation, I would offer an excuse that became a running joke. I would say, "There's not enough parking where you live; I'm not coming."

Reflecting on this, a more honest answer would have been, "No way! I look frightening in a swimsuit. Why would I hang out at the beach?"

Thank goodness my friends ignored my excuses and continued to extend invitations. Being truly wonderful people, they would often create a parking spot just for me.

Since that time, I have seen old photos of myself wearing a swimsuit, and my body didn't look as awful as I had imagined. My overly visual perspective, plus my embarrassment with my body image had created these negative perceptions.

I decided that I wanted to discover as much as I could about my undirected wants. The thoughts log explored those emotions that connected body image with food taste. These thoughts caused me to cheat and stop exercising. Time and time again, I had become distracted by my inability to control past memories. These negative thoughts interrupted my weight loss by redirecting my focus to influential emotions stored in my subconscious. I realized that by identifying which thoughts caused me to overeat, I could control my reactions to certain foods.

In recent years a trip to the beach is no longer a threatening experience, and wearing a swimsuit has not been unbearable.

I also discovered that undirected wants take time to identify, and after they have been identified, more time is needed to find and practice replacement thoughts.

A World of Imbalance

Undirected wants live in the unconscious mind. When they resurface, they cause me to overeat, sleep less, and make bad menu decisions. The influence they carry is so subtle that it can interrupt weight loss and stop the diet altogether.

Any kind of food distraction can result from undirected wants. This could be something as simple as eating a chocolate bar in the afternoon when there is a lull in energy. Stating the obvious, the chocolate bar is often not part of the diet, and this sort of unconscious eating is usually triggered by a sensory reaction to boredom or as a response to a highly charged emotional situation.

Undirected wants have also caused me to overeat both in secret and alone. The memories span as long ago as my childhood, when I ate meals in my bedroom, to as recently as a few years ago, when I decided to eat decadent foods that I loved while being alone at home.

These undirected wants can be difficult to identify because they may be connected to recurring events and a multitude of emotions. These particular emotions are distinguishable because they cause us to eat special, high-calorie foods.

It soon became clear that undirected wants had prevented me from reaching my weight loss goal. If I could not identify them, then I would continue to hang on to these memories like a favorite stuffed toy. If I did lose weight during these cycles, this weight would return, and so would the habit of yo-yo dieting.

It was surprising to learn that even after I established new positive thoughts, undirected wants continued to affect how I made food decisions. This reinforced how critical awareness and identification were to the entire weight loss process.

As previously mentioned, I noticed that many of my undirected wants had recurring themes, such as the need to feel included. An example of one of these themes has two parts. When replayed, part one sounds something like this: "I want to order the same amazing dessert that my friend ordered." Part two of this conversation is not spoken but thought: "It's okay to have dessert; when I exercise tomorrow, I will burn off the extra calories."

To prevent any further impact, I began to use the Do Monkey support tools to develop a creative thinking environment. This environment allowed me to rely on solutions and new thoughts, which moved me through moments of diet uncertainty so I could make healthier food choices.

Replacing Undirected Wants

Not knowing how many undirected wants I had, the only way to achieve control over these thoughts was to continue the process of identification. This practice also helped to isolate the role of certain food tastes that were connected to relationships with other people and certain events in my life.

As it relates to a congregation of memories—for example, the need to fit in with others—I have replaced these particular undirected wants with new thoughts and food associations, which are focused on building better relationships.

Monkey Survival

The Weight Loss Monkeys do not have undirected wants.

Indeed, most animals are not affected by extreme bouts of emotion because they have fewer complex thoughts. They also do not have the same emotional reactions to food as humans. Their main reason for eating food is elemental; it is to survive.

In contrast, people have a spectrum of complex emotions that nurture a thinking environment in which undirected wants collect and can be recalled. They are expressed through unrealized thoughts, which resurface frequently and without our conscious awareness.

Under these conditions, food is used to reestablish the order that has been created by recurring negative emotions. Any resulting weight gain serves to disguise our past hurts, and then it no longer matters what, why, or when food is being eaten.

Monkey Reaction

Having less emotional expression, monkeys and other wild animals tend to focus on using food to replenish their overall physical strength. This promotes their ability to produce the creative responses necessary to manage their natural habitats. This also makes eating a healthy diet critical to their survival and the subsequent evolution of their species.

In contrast, primitive threats to human survival have virtually been removed from urban living, and the control mechanisms in our brains have adapted to less threatening environments. These subdued mind conditions have resulted in an unconscious reduction of physical movement, which is a natural component to weight management.

Both the dieter and health advocate have bodies that have become weakened as a result of a lack of natural exercise and good nutrition. This overall physical weakness makes them susceptible to emotion-rich thoughts that are connected to certain "special" foods.

Under the influence of undirected wants, yo-yo dieting becomes frequent, particularly when we continue to have poor weight loss results. In addition, terminating diets without reaching the goal ensures only one thing, that there will be more weight gain in the future.

Within this ideology, the need for survival is viewed as the counter-reaction to the undirected want. During the weight loss program, when the key focus becomes survival as a means of improving health, the undirected wants become less influential and weaken over time.

Survival of the Fittest

Successful food management depends on the ability to reduce and eliminate undirected wants. This can be accomplished by reinstating the survival instinct.

Both visits to the doctor and being aware of our health can produce a greater survival instinct, which in turn supports a greater health focus.

Monkey Questions: Reasoning

The answers to the following questions identify undirected wants.

- Why do you want to lose weight and get healthy?
- Why do you want to start a new diet?
- Are there past food thoughts that you are still connected to? What are they?
- Are these thoughts about specific foods, events, or people? List all of these thoughts and their associations.
- Are there certain "special" foods that you eat often? List these foods.

- How can you pay better attention to your feelings when you eat these "special" foods?

Monkey Chapter Summary

Undirected wants are responsible for sabotaging weight loss. They survive as a congregation of negative thought emotions, which are created by the mind and survive through past memories.

Undirected wants have increased influence when there are limited threats to survival.

The impact of undirected wants can be minimized by having a deeper understanding of our physical health and creating a greater survival instinct.

~ ~ ~

Monkey Chapter Notes

Chapter Seven

How Much Weight to Lose?

Weight Stages

In the past, my health objectives have been based on unrealistic expectations. Even at age forty-something, I still clung to a fabricated illusion of what my body image should look like. This image was connected to weight loss ideals that were based on numbers taken from what is commonly referred to as the height and weight tables of the Metropolitan Life Insurance Company, 1983. This chart is still used by several popular diets as a suggested weight range guide for adults.[3]

During previous diet attempts, when I had achieved significant weight loss, I remember feeling fabulous, my clothes fitting well, and exercise being more manageable. Unfortunately, this euphoria was always fleeting. I would gain back the weight when I became disconnected and unfocused with my goal.

Logically, I understood that each diet worked, because I had lost weight. Even the food routines I created worked. What had not worked had been my ability to reach a significant weight loss milestone, remain focused, and stay at that weight.

Consistent use of all the Monkey tools helped me to produce greater health awareness, and this in turn changed my weight loss goal.

There were three rules I used to arrive at this new goal. First, I had to make sure that I fully embraced my new health focus. Second, the goal could not be associated with any emotional thoughts that could be triggered by specific tastes. Last, this number had to represent a weight range that I could manage for a lifetime.

Monkey Dieter Belief System

Having a realistic and attainable weight loss goal is the foundation of the Monkey Dieter Belief System. When the goal is attainable, motivation becomes easier to sustain.

Motivation can improve diet behaviors by increasing awareness. A motivation-driven belief system reduces the impact of negative emotions and maintains a positive dieting environment.

Mapping Out the Vision

During the first phase of my health initiative, I recorded my weight every day. These numbers included body weight, water fluctuations, and changes in fat. Scales that easily compute these calculations can be purchased that are not too expensive and are readily available. Once I had accumulated enough information, approximately three months of data, I could better understand how much weight I could lose in a specific period of time and at certain metabolic thresholds.

I also decided to find out what my body shape might look like when I reached my goal weight. During previous weight loss experiences, my body image ideal had been based on perceptions of other people's body shapes. These unrealistic views only served to create disappointment, particularly when the reading on the scale never matched my true physical proportions.

Monkey Action

Make a label with your new weight loss goal and affix this label to your weight scale. This number is your customized weight loss goal. The label represents a daily visual reminder of the final destination in your personal weight loss journey.

Monkey Questions: The New Goal

Write a detailed response to each of these questions. Use numbers as an expression of the weight you want to lose.

- In a perfect world, what do you want to weigh and why?
- Is this number realistic given your weight loss history?
- Does this number make sense based on your age and the efficiency of your metabolism?
- What reasonable and safe amount of weight loss can you accomplish so that you can feel better and stay motivated? Write down a number between one and five pounds.
- Answer these questions again in ninety days. Add this date to your calendar and compare your answers based on the

weight you have actually lost. If necessary, after ninety days has passed, answer the next questions. Be specific and honest. Remember, no one will see these answers except for you.

- Why have you not lost as much weight as you expected to lose?
- What part of your health plan needs to be adjusted to ensure you lose weight in a more efficient manner?
- Could your slow weight loss be health-related? Do you need to make an appointment with your doctor to get more information?

The Weight Loss Tracking Tool

Review the sample weight loss tracking tool (see Figure 2) and then create your own customized version.

The weight loss tracking tool can be used to track both efficient and poor periods of weight loss. It can also monitor unusual fluctuations in weight, as well as water retention.

By adding a note section to your tracking tool, you will be able to monitor unusual food events and any changes you make in your diet plan.

Monkey Questions: Focus Improves Motivation

Write one short paragraph for each of these questions.

- What can you do today to improve your health focus?
- Are these new ideas something you can realistically maintain?

- What additional changes in your diet and exercise routine can you make to improve your weight loss results?
- Could any of these new changes interrupt your focus?
- What can you do to deter negative thoughts so that you can stay on your plan?

The Monkey Factor

The Monkey factor is the dieter's personal weight loss desire, which is supported by a statement.

The Monkey factor represents the dieter's most important reason to lose weight.

Becoming aware of the Monkey factor produces sustained motivation and improves weight loss. The purpose of having sustained motivation is to discourage diet lapses and unconscious eating.

How to Create Your Monkey Factor

Each dieter will have his or her own reason to lose weight.

To identify this reason, answer the following question.

If there are several reasons for weight loss, take a moment to rank each reason in order of importance.* The reason that is your number-one weight loss priority will be your Monkey factor.

What are your Monkey factors?

1. ____

____

____

2. ____

____

____

3. ____

____

____

4. ____

____

____

5. ____

____

____

*Remember, if there is more than one, rank each factor in order of importance.

Monkey Chapter Summary

The final weight loss goal can be customized.

Creating an accurate weight loss goal, and combining this with your true metabolic efficiency and ideal body image, can produce motivation and greater weight loss focus.

The Monkey factor represents the true reason the dieter will implement the diet or health initiative.

~ ~ ~

Weight Loss Tracking Tool

Date	Weight	Fat	Water	Food Plan Changes/ Comments

Figure 2. Weight Loss Tracking Tool (Make Copies)

Weight Loss Tracking Tool Instructions

Weigh daily to chart progress and identify water fluctuations. The goal is to understand how the body loses weight over a specific period of time. In the short term, because of fluctuations (up and down), this may seem to be a frustrating process. However, after collecting enough data, this tracking tool can provide important and helpful information that identifies progress and addresses any adjustments that may be required to improve weight loss results.

Weight Chart for Women

From height and weight tables of the Metropolitan Life Insurance Company, 1983.
Weight in pounds, based on ages 25–59 with the lowest mortality rate (indoor clothing weighing 3 pounds and shoes with 1-inch heels).

Height in Shoes	Small Frame	Medium Frame	Large Frame
6'	138 to 151	148 to 162	158 to 179
5'11"	135 to 148	145 to 159	155 to 176
5'10"	132 to 145	142 to 156	152 to 173
5'9"	129 to 142	139 to 153	149 to 170
5'8"	126 to 139	136 to 150	146 to 167
5'7"	123 to 136	133 to 147	143 to 163
5'6"	120 to 133	130 to 144	140 to 159
5'5"	117 to 130	127 to 141	137 to 155
5'4"	114 to 127	124 to 138	134 to 151
5'3"	111 to 124	121 to 135	131 to 147
5'2"	108 to 121	118 to 132	128 to 143
5'1"	106 to 118	115 to 129	125 to 140
5'	104 to 115	113 to 126	122 to 137
4'11"	103 to 113	111 to 123	120 to 134
4'10"	102 to 111	109 to 121	118 to 131

Weight Chart for Men

Weight in pounds, based on ages 25–59 with the lowest mortality rate (indoor clothing weighing 5 pounds and shoes with 1-inch heels).

Height in Shoes	Small Frame	Medium Frame	Large Frame
6'4"	162 to 176	171 to 187	181 to 207
6'3"	158 to 172	167 to 182	176 to 202
6'2"	155 to 168	164 to 178	172 to 197
6'1"	152 to 164	160 to 174	168 to 192
6'	149 to 160	157 to 170	164 to 188
5'11"	146 to 157	154 to 166	161 to 184
5'10"	144 to 154	151 to 163	158 to 180
5'9"	142 to 151	148 to 160	155 to 176
5'8"	140 to 148	145 to 157	152 to 172
5'7"	138 to 145	142 to 154	149 to 168
5'6"	136 to 142	139 to 151	146 to 164
5'5"	134 to 140	137 to 148	144 to 160
5'4"	132 to 138	135 to 145	142 to 156
5'3"	130 to 136	133 to 143	140 to 153
5'2"	128 to 134	131 to 141	138 to 150

Monkey Chapter Notes

How Much Weight to Lose?

Chapter Eight

Use the Monkey Tools

Weighty Obstacles

Weighing myself represented the continuous use of one particular diet tool, the scales. This particular tool symbolized a daily visual reminder of my actual weight.

Weighing myself was often a frustrating experience, which could produce not only negative thoughts but excuses to eat more food. Every time I got on the scale, I wished the numbers were smaller. Unfortunately, these perceptions were unrealistic based on the efficiency of my metabolism, the chosen food plan, and the amount of exercise I had committed to.

Weight gain also produced bouts of mild depression, which could lead to taste triggers and eventually ending the diet.

Scale Power

During one of these unfocused diet moments, I had the not-so-brilliant idea of putting my scale in storage.

This proved to be a huge mistake. I gained weight, lots of weight, more than thirty pounds. I hadn't noticed the weight or my clothes sizes going up. Without seeing the numbers on the scale, I had lost that all-important visual connection with my body image. Not having the scale also served to make me vulnerable to negative food thoughts and the emotions that caused me to overeat.

Today, I consider my scales—yes, I use two—as the most beneficial "See" support tool. I record my weight loss (and gain) on a daily log, and I weigh myself every morning.

I noticed periods of weight gain, particularly during monthly hormone fluctuations. However, because I had recorded my daily weight, I knew exactly how much of this weight was water retention and how this water retention could impact my diet focus.

These numbers also identified exactly how much weight my body could lose and in what period of time. Having this information produced a new focus; I could pinpoint when I had reached a weight loss plateau. When these plateaus happened, I could re-evaluate both my eating and exercise routines and make adjustments.

When the numbers on the scale were positive, this encouraged mini celebrations. My new reward system (at five-pound milestones) included planned events, a movie date, or some other social experience with other people.

Monkey Chapter Summary

The scale, when used continuously, is the tool that can gather weight loss information and also monitor emotional eating.

Daily weigh-ins identify weight fluctuations, track both weight lost and weight gained, and support the importance of using motivational tools.

The scale is considered a visual tool that monitors more than just weight; it also monitors the dieter's level of weight loss enthusiasm.

~ ~ ~

Monkey Chapter Notes

Use the Monkey Tools

Chapter Nine

Visual Appeal

A Self-portrait

Improving food observations resulted in making better menu choices. I became interested in how foods were prepared, their attractiveness, and most important, how the look of food impacted my undirected wants.

Because my mind connected memories to certain foods, this new awareness changed how I participated in visually rich food experiences. Examples include popular holiday events such as Thanksgiving and Easter, and vacations to places where food was inexpensive and readily available.

Monkey Questions: The Looker

Write a short paragraph response to each of the following questions.

- Do you believe smaller portions look satisfying, and if so, why?

- Do certain foods look more attractive than others? List these foods.
- When you weigh less on the scale, do you look smaller? If you don't look smaller, does this bother you and why?
- When you are dieting, do you visualize celery, carrots, and vegetables as yummy treats? If not, why not?
- What visual reminders can you use to help you become more diet conscious, particularly at social events where your special foods are served?
- List any upcoming food events in your life and how you will make food choices during these events. (This question should be answered once a month and used as a planning tool for occasions that are focused around food.)
- What are your favorite desserts?
- Why did you choose the desserts on your list (was it because of taste, flavor, or memory)?
- How often do you eat dessert?
- How important is eating desserts and sweet foods? Find out after tracking a full week of eating.
- What do you think would happen to you if you ate fewer desserts?
- How many desserts and sweets do you think you can eliminate during the next week? Write down a number and stick to it!

How Others View Food

Companies that sell prepared foods as part of their diet programs understand the value of visual appeal. These foods may taste awful, but they have to look appetizing, particularly when presented as part of a marketing, advertising or sales promotion.

If the dieter selects one of these options for weight loss, greater focus is required to avoid eating the trigger foods that are part of the planned menu and that may encourage negative food emotions.

In each case, prepared meals are considered fictional foods that offer temporary emotional distractions.

Monkey Questions: The Yummy Factor

List all the foods you love.

- Do you have any memory connections with these foods?
- Describe some of these memories. When was the first time you ever ate these foods?
- Search your photo albums for visual food events. Examine these pictures closely. Are there any foods that are memorable? When was the last time you ate these specific foods?
- When you visualize the foods you love, what sensory taste characteristics stand out? Sensory examples include sweet, sour, or salty. List these foods with their corresponding sensory taste connections. Rank them in order of taste importance, one being the most important.
- How many times in your life have you eaten these foods?
- Why do you continue to eat these foods when you have eaten them many times before?
- What foods can be used to substitute your "special" foods? These replacement foods must be satisfying and palatable.

~ ~ ~

Monkey Chapter Notes

Visual Appeal

Chapter Ten

Who Am I? Image Identification

Body Shapes

A point of frustration was being unable to predict what my body would look like after my weight was comfortably managed. It was also true that how I looked when I was age nine and healthy could not be replicated in my mid-forties. Another issue was whether I would be satisfied with a new and unfamiliar body image.

Repeating daily body shape affirmations produced answers to these concerns. It became clear that only a new focus and staying on my diet plan could result in acceptance of this new me. My fears about body shape had been born out of my subconscious, using a file folder of memories that were no longer useful, and had kept me in a comfortable state of obesity.

The first step was to use the Monkey tools—writing, tracking, and using affirmations to stabilize my focus. After my weight goal was achieved, I recognized that I was now a smaller, lighter person and how much more I liked myself that way.

Here's Looking at You!

In 2005, I attended an amazing workshop about identifying people's characteristics through sensory awareness. I was surprised to discover that I evaluated my life and body image from a visual perspective.

This is not unusual since as a collective society we tend to gravitate toward various forms of visual media such as television, the Internet, and magazines, which continue to influence how we think.

Being highly visual, I based the majority of my decisions on how I saw life. Appearance, particularly my own, mattered. How food looked meant more to me than how it tasted. With such a huge emphasis on the visual, I realized that better health and self-love would be difficult to achieve if I never discovered which visual images impacted my food decisions.

Tool by Tool

As this evaluation process continued, my health initiative found a new level of enthusiasm. Weighing myself became a ritual of self-appreciation, and the scales became my new best friend.

I also discovered that not all of my visual perspectives were negative. The one tool that became a significant source of encouragement was the Monkey tracing tool, which I used to create a blueprint of my desired body image.

Using both childhood and recent photos of myself, I was able to design a template of my body shape, which created a "before" and "after" weight loss impression. This tool produced a greater appreciation for what I could look like after I had reached my weight loss goal.

To create these impressions, I chose photos of my body image before I had weight issues. At age nine, I was a child with a normal amount of body fat. It was surprising to discover that the basic silhouette of my body image had not changed over the years. Even at age nine, my legs were thick, my waist small, and I had a natural pear shape.

I have to admit that it was difficult to identify with that nine-year-old. I couldn't even recall a single memory of that time in my life. This made me realize how far in the past my undirected wants had had influence.

I decided to view my tracing often and taped the sketch onto my computer monitor.

To increase my level of motivation, each day I would hold the sketch and repeat the following statements:

- I appreciate my true body shape.
- This picture represents my true physical self, the one that does not rely on food.
- This image of myself is happy in every way.
- This image of myself is not associated with any food connected to emotional pain created in my past.

Monkey Instructions: Tracing Tool

You will need:

- 2 sheets of tracing paper or kitchen wax paper
- A black pencil
- A colored pencil
- 2 pictures. One of your best body image ever. The other, a recent picture of yourself that is not older than 10 days.

The goal is to create a final drawing or visual impression of your desired body shape. See Figure 3 for example.

Using a sheet of tracing paper, trace your desired body image using the old photo. On the other sheet of tracing paper, trace your current body image. This will result in two tracings, one image larger in proportion to the other.

For each sketch, draw strong, bold lines of the body silhouette. This will make the lines on each tracing appear clearly imprinted. **Note**: The size of each frame may be skewed based on the pictures you have chosen, which may vary by age, height, and body size.

Place the ideal (desired) body image tracing under the current body image tracing and copy the outline of this image using the colored pencil. One sheet will overlap the other; the imprint of the ideal body image will be transferred onto (or into) the larger body image tracing.

This final drawing will identify which areas of your body can be toned by using a combination of proper diet and exercise.

The tracing tool can be repeated at various stages of weight loss. To repeat the process, you will need to have updated pictures of your body after you reach each weight loss milestone.

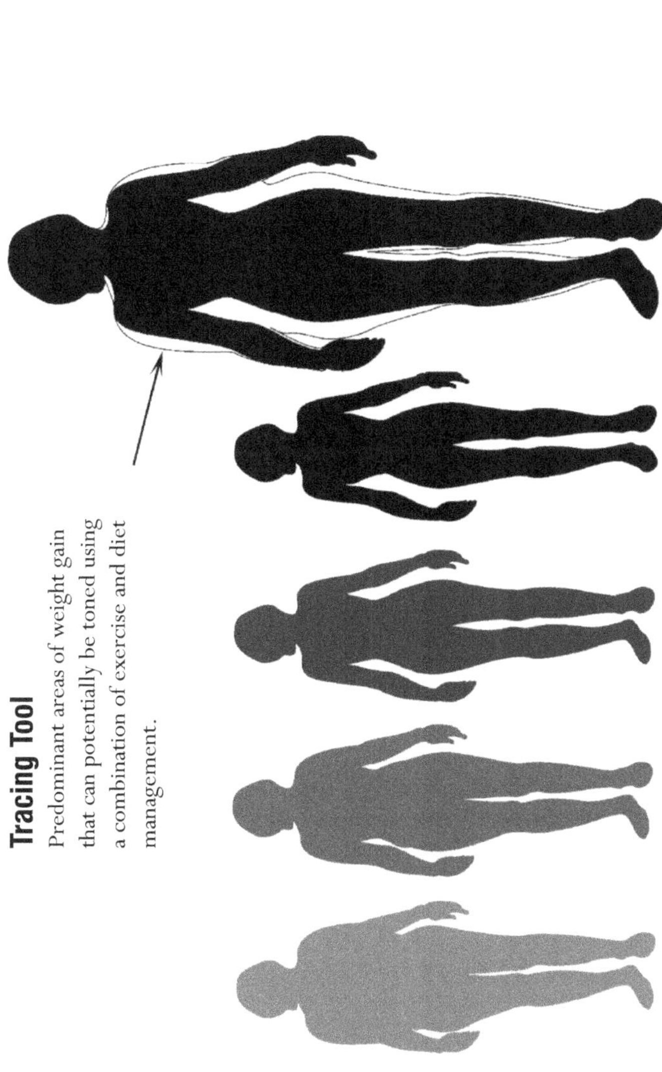

Figure 3. Change in body size from largest to smallest frame. These silhouettes can be created by tracing the outlines of older and newer photos of the dieter's body image to identify a new, desired body shape.

Monkey Chapter Summary

The combined use of motivation and the tracing tool improves the flow of positive thoughts. Frequent use of these tools can help to reshape the dieter's visual perspective by creating a more realistic future body image.

~ ~ ~

Monkey Chapter Notes

Monkey Say

Chapter Eleven

Directed Wants

"Most creatures who roam our earth are completely free of resistance. In contrast, humans are able to focus their thoughts in deliberate ways, and in doing so can create more resistance than they are aware of."

—Unknown author

Say Monkey Tools

Directed wants improve the dieter's ability to focus.

Using the following Say Monkey tools produces the motivation necessary to support greater weight loss. These tools also elevate the importance of the dieter's primary Monkey factor, his or her main reason for wanting to lose weight or to become healthy.

Monkey Mind

Affirmations and meditation are the primary Say Monkey tools. When used regularly, they increase positive thoughts and diet focus.

After I introduced the practice of daily affirmations, my overall health awareness improved, and this installed a framework of creative weight loss ideas. Instilling more positive thoughts also helped to produce the level of enthusiasm I needed to maintain my health initiative.

Decades of collecting unhealthy food thoughts had produced behaviors that sabotaged each diet. Continuing on this unhealthy path also ensured that I would ignore the emotional pain that was the underlying cause of my overeating.

The affirmations I created were customized so that they mirrored my weight loss goals. They were designed specifically to restore my poor self-image and to identify how this self-image negatively impacted my relationships with other people. These relationships included interactions with friends, family members, acquaintances, colleagues, and even business associates.

Having a raised consciousness served to make me aware of the influences of my negative thoughts. These thoughts could control which clothes I purchased, how much I exercised, and most important, how reclusive and less social I became when I gained weight.

Restraining the influence of negative food thoughts required that I use these Monkey tools every day.

The affirmation tool, in particular, created the type of awareness I needed so that I could become more outgoing. Of course, these changes didn't happen overnight; it took continuous practice.

I never realized how much I avoided social interactions until my food behaviors became health directed. Having this added focus allowed me to relax and enjoy the company of other people without worrying what I was going to eat next.

Practicing Affirmations

I would repeat my affirmations out loud with my hand on my chest (similar to our actions when we say the American Pledge of Allegiance). This hand position increases the power of the affirmation, as it connects to the natural vibration resonating from the body. With regular use, the sound energy creates a new, positive thought environment.

Affirmations also can be recited in silence, but this is not as effective because the absence of the sound vibration delays the installation of the positive thought.

I customized each statement so that it would compliment my new health initiative, while at the same time produce new, positive eating behaviors.

I repeated each affirmation out loud during long walks. These days, I'm not too embarrassed when passersby hear me speak them out loud.

The first realization that I had while assimilating these new thoughts came as a pleasant surprise. This happened when I noticed that I avoided certain "special" foods that I normally gravitated toward. Positive food responses also signaled that the influence of my undirected wants had weakened.

Monkey Instructions: Creating Affirmations

The majority of affirmations should be created using "I" statements.

Using the word I as part of the affirmation establishes a personal responsibility for the new food behaviors.

There is no limit to the number of positive "I" affirmations that can be created.

Repetition is the key to producing faster results, while at the same time accelerating the installation of the new thought environment. To encourage this process, it is recommended that the affirmations be repeated three or more times in succession. This continuous repetition establishes the new thought and associated behaviors.

Affirmation Example

Condition: I eat too many chocolates and sweets.
Affirmation: I am chocolate free.

~ ~ ~

More Sample Affirmations

- I am thin.
- I am a size ____.
- I weigh ____ pounds.
- I am an example of glorious good health.
- I lead a more active life.
- I enjoy exercise every day.

~ ~ ~

List your top three Monkey factors (described in Chapter 7).

1. ______

2. ______

3. ______

Using your Monkey factors, construct your customized affirmations using "I" statements.

1. ______

2. ______

3. ______

4. ______

5. ______

6. ____

____

7. ____

____

8. ____

____

9. ____

____

10. ____

____

Monkey Meditation: Creating Stillness

Why does a positive health focus require stillness?

Mind stillness produces the space to create positive food thoughts. Mind stillness also improves awareness of negative food thoughts that are connected to memories and replayed in continuous cycles.

Meditation—How It Works

Where affirmations complement positive thought vibrations, meditation creates the stillness that helps to restore the dieter's ability to produce productive food behaviors.

Because we have so many thoughts, complete mind silence is next to impossible to achieve. A mind that takes advantage of stillness and ignores everyday distractions is better able to produce increased positive thoughts.

Monkey meditation does not require hours or days; Monkey meditation requires only seconds.

The beginner's goal is thirty seconds of no thoughts every day. This will require some practice. A goal of thirty seconds without thought or zero thoughts is not easy to achieve, so be patient with this tool.

This thirty-second practice can be incorporated into any convenient moment of your day. To build the practice, continue to add additional thirty-second intervals.

Expanding this tool, Monkey meditation can extend beyond thirty seconds to many minutes of mind stillness. Remember, this is a practice and requires patience to master.

Creative Edge

The purpose of continuous mind stillness is to introduce periods of creative thinking, which encourages new ideas that are focused on improving good health.

Many of our thoughts about food are formed because we repeat unconscious eating behaviors. These behaviors impair our ability to be creative. Examples include eating the same breakfast every day, choosing the same sandwich, or returning to age-old food habits after the diet has ended.

In contrast, directed wants produce creative diet ideas that support the new weight loss goal. As the dieter's awareness improves, new behaviors emerge. Examples include preparing salads with different vegetables or switching decadent foods with healthy substitutes.

The positive proof of these changes can only be fully appreciated with regular use of these practices.

Meditation Instructions

Monkey meditation increases its effectiveness when it is exercised in quiet surroundings. Do not attempt Monkey meditation in a moving vehicle or in noisy, crowded areas.

You will need a comfortable place to sit or lie down.

Part I

Inhale through the nose and exhale through the mouth. These are continuous, slow, gentle, and deep breaths. Repeat this practice as often as time permits. The first goal is to continue these deep breaths for thirty seconds.

Part II

After the cycle is complete, take a few moments to focus and "listen" to your body. An example of this includes the rhythm of your heartbeat or the sound of your breathing. Do your best not to think about the rhythm of your heartbeat or sound of your breathing; instead, focus on the actual actions. Other sensory examples include the movement of your lips, the texture of your mouth and the temperature of your breath.

Monkey Chapter Summary

Combining meditation and positive affirmations as a daily practice produces a mind state in which negative food thoughts have less influence.

A positive and focused thought environment reduces food cravings, introduces creative food ideas, and helps to maintain the integrity of the diet or the health initiative.

~ ~ ~

Monkey Chapter Notes

Directed Wants

Chapter Twelve

Which Diet to Choose?

A Self-portrait

Over the years, my choice in diets has alternated between popular trends and fads—the most important criterion being my level of desperation at the time the choice was being made.

My favorite type of diet was commonly referred to as "high protein." I enjoyed being on these programs, not because I had a deep-rooted appreciation for meat and animal byproducts, but because these diets were convenient and required no portion control. I could easily eat a burger omitting the bun or attend social functions without feeling awkward or deprived when vegetables and chicken were offered.

I had known people who had lost weight on these high-protein programs; however, I never had the same results. After trying several of these plans, I noticed that the efficiency of my digestion changed for the worse. The lack of fiber alone served to slow my metabolism to a point where it could not be returned to normal.

Also, my body and taste sensations preferred sugary foods and carbohydrates, so eliminating these foods for extended periods only created uncontrollable cravings.

In addition, based on my diet history, I had never been consistent. A lifetime of poor diet vigilance would guarantee that regardless of which plan I chose, my negative thoughts would not allow me to reach my weight goal.

The Monkey tools became vital to the success of my overall process. The thoughts log produced greater awareness of my negative food behaviors. The regular use of affirmations and meditation resulted in creative solutions, particularly during periods of food boredom when I needed more diet focus.

Old Food Behaviors

A review of my thoughts log identified that there were three recurring behaviors that continued to interrupt my diet progress. First, I had never stayed on any plan long enough to reach my weight loss goal. Second, I had never arrived at a point where I could maintain the weight I had lost. Finally, during all of those years of dieting, I had never made a permanent lifestyle change. In fact, diet consistency had always been a problem; one week I was high protein, the next vegetarian, then sometime after that I tried being vegan, and so on. Eventually I would eat meat again.

All the diets of the past had revolved around temporary practices, and I would eventually resume eating the same foods I had enjoyed in the past as soon as I became bored of the diet.

The Basic Plan

In recent years, marketing for the diet industry has become more sophisticated. However, it still surprises me that the main premise for most diets has not changed. Either they introduce tasty foods and recipes or they promote plans that distribute how calories are consumed.

After years of yo-yo dieting, achieving results, and then failing, I realized that desperation was no longer an acceptable reason for being on any plan. I had to focus on finding ways to eat high-quality foods and to stay on just one program.

I understood that most of the commercial diets could result in some level of success; however, in each case all the rules had to be applied to achieve the goal and then to maintain the weight loss.

Choosing the Final Diet

As previously discussed, undirected wants take the typical dieter out of weight loss focus. In contrast, establishing directed wants stimulates focus by improving how we creatively think about food, weight loss, and health management.

Choosing the correct diet also relies on our ability to fully commit to the food plan. Cheating, making diet modifications, not exercising, and deviating from the basic instructions are all signs of a diminished diet focus, which eventually leads to poor weight loss results and the possibility of complete diet failure.

Staying power, rather than modified eating, becomes more important to the final outcome. Also, the health plan chosen must be one that can be managed and augmented over time to accommodate social interactions with food. This permanent plan can never be replaced, even when new diets are introduced.

Those who have successfully managed their weight for a lifetime do so because they have created a customized plan that supports their overall health and can be practiced for a lifetime.

The Monkey Diets

Since most health books about diets are expected to include a nutrition plan, the Weight Loss Monkeys have included two options designed to embrace the motivational ideas discussed in this book. The main premise is that most diets work. Unfortunately, a diet will not be effective unless the dieter has a full understanding of his or her existing beliefs about the role of food, the body image desired, and making those necessary lifestyle changes that will achieve optimum health.

~ ~ ~

The Weight Loss Monkeys (and I) are not doctors or nutritionists. Please make sure that any diet you select in the future has been approved by your physician.

~ ~ ~

The following Monkey food plans do not advocate drastic changes but a gradual inclusion of high-quality foods. As a reminder, during the first diet stage, enthusiasm propels success. However, the impact of taste and past emotions can influence the dieter's food wants and needs, and this is what will eventually impair diet focus.

The Diet: A Word or Two More

As most of you know, there are thousands of diets on the market, but accomplishing the goal will require a high degree of focus.

The following Monkey diet programs offer a starting point for understanding better health and nutrition.

Remember, diets are always temporary unless you make the results permanent.

Monkey Focus

As you read about these diets, pay close attention to your thoughts. Write these perspectives in your thoughts log. Also, how do you rate these perspectives? Are they positive or negative?

Ten Fingers Gorilla Overview

The dieter or health enthusiast may not be ready to start a formal diet. The Ten Fingers Gorilla Plan provides the beginning steps towards a new health initiative. This is achieved by gradually building new health behaviors.

In the absence of a formal diet plan, more focus will be required because there will be much more to think about. More thoughts always require more creative actions.

Ten Fingers Gorilla Plan

TIME—Eating based not on clock time but actual hunger. Also, the right amount of time for food preparation and exercise.

ETERNAL—A plan used anytime, anyplace, anywhere.

NOW—Improved mind health and focus using the Monkey tools.

FREE—70–80 percent colorful foods. Increase fruit and vegetable intake and avoid all-white foods like sugar, flour, and salt.

IRRIGATE—Water: enough to completely hydrate the body every day.

NATURAL—No foods with hormones, pesticides, antibiotics, additives, pills, potions, or chemicals.

GROWN—Actual foods; eat nothing artificial.

ENERGY—Exercise enough to stay mobile, be fit, and maintain a desired weight range.

ROUTINE—Meal management. When and how often we eat food.

STRIVE—Creative ideas to limit diet boredom. Examples include taking food preparation classes and experimenting with new recipes.

Supplementation

Daily use of the Monkey tools and unlimited entries in the thoughts log. Other useful Monkey support tools including meditation and affirmations.

Vitamins as needed. Check with your doctor for the correct dosage.

Exercise as much as is safe and reasonable.

~ ~ ~

Always check with your doctor
before starting any new diet or health plan!

Chimpanzee Plan Overview

Chimps are usually uninhibited, adapt to change, and can follow instructions. Similar to smaller monkeys, the Chimpanzee Plan has been designed to promote freedom of mobility. The Chimpanzee Plan adopts the use of commercial health plans and diets.

Chimpanzee Plan

The dieter picks the diet he or she wants.

Important: Pick a diet that you like and that you can manage for a lifetime.

Monkey Note

Try to avoid unusually high protein diets. Keep in mind, eating sufficient fiber is a natural component of maintaining good health. Eliminating protein requires more digestion efficiency. Because these plans usually lack sufficient fiber, drinking enough water is vital to aiding digestion and elimination.

Supplementation

Daily use of the Monkey tools and unlimited entries in the thoughts log. Other useful Monkey support tools including meditation and affirmations.

Vitamins as needed. Check with your doctor for the correct dosage.

Exercise as much as is safe and reasonable.

Remember to write down your thoughts about these two programs.

~ ~ ~

Always check with your doctor
before starting any new diet or health plan!

Monkey Chapter Summary

When choosing a diet, consider how a lifetime of unhealthy eating has hurt your weight loss progress.

There are unknown risks associated with eating chemicals, growth hormones, pesticides, and bulk derivatives, which already exist in our foods and diet supplements.

The Weight Loss Monkeys encourage a focused diet approach that recognizes the importance of eating naturally grown foods.

Eliminating processed food from our diet is both important and necessary to improving long-term health and avoiding future health risks.

Eating foods that are not in their purest forms also creates unknown food distractions such as bingeing, overeating, and complex digestion issues. The purer the foods, the fewer the distractions, the more focused the diet results will be, the greater the weight loss, and the fewer the risks to our overall health.

~ ~ ~

Monkey Chapter Notes

Chapter Thirteen

People Distractions

A Self-portrait

Watching and participating in the eating habits of others impacted how I gained and lost weight.

I discovered that there are two primary groups of eaters whose food behaviors mattered to me. The largest group is composed of mainstream eaters, who use food to elevate their dining experiences by focusing on taste. As far as mainstream eaters are concerned, the choice of restaurant and the menu decisions really don't matter.

The second group is the most influential when it comes to weight loss. This group is divided into two subgroups, the food mentors and the alternative eaters. Food mentors are distinguished by their use of food as a tool. They never discuss weight issues because they are always focused on their health. Food mentors are also influenced by a different set of undirected wants that are contrary to taste. When it comes to food decisions, they always ignore social norms and make food choices that are focused on better health and nutrition.

In my late forties, I made the decision to find my own food mentors. These were people whom I could talk to about food and any health-related issues including diet and exercise.

Finding the right individuals to be my food mentors proved to be an interesting and long-range project. This experience taught me that most of the people in my existing food circle practiced mostly mainstream eating habits.

Eater Distinctions

One of the primary distractions for most dieters is being surrounded by mainstream eaters. The majority of mainstream eaters enjoy all types of food, particularly those decadent foods that are viewed as unhealthy.

Mainstream eaters cannot do without coffee, tea, soda, or chocolate; they do not avoid commercial foods; they often rely on medications; and they consider exercise not a habit but a chore.

It surprised me that very few of my friends even came close to being a true food mentor. In fact, when I was reviewing my selection process, I discovered that almost all of my friends participated in at least one mainstream behavior. This created a new category of health-conscious individuals, whom I describe as alternative eaters. This group is equally health focused; they still participate in modified mainstream eating but practice portion control and expend more calories because they participate in vigorous exercise.

I realized that when it came to the important subject of my health, I had to focus on adopting an alternative eating approach. I realized that mainstream eating would always be influential and that everyday food distractions would continue to be a big part of my life. It was now up to me to take responsibility for not only what I ate but also whom I ate with.

If almost everyone I met was a mainstream eater, then I had to make sure that the individuals I spent the most time with were alternative eaters. These individuals were focused on making better health decisions and, more often than not, ate mostly high-quality foods.

Being on any diet also required choosing companions who offered motivation and support during the weight loss process and beyond.

Monkey Chapter Summary

Because there are so many food choices, there will always be a predominance of mainstream eaters who often participate in unfocused eating and avoid exercise.

The final weight loss and health outcome relies not only on how we manage our diets but also which people we surround ourselves with, particularly during soscial dining experiences.

The dieter may enjoy the company of a mixture of both mainstream and alternative eaters; however, traditional food mentors are the most successful food, diet, and weight managers.

~ ~ ~

Monkey Chapter Notes

People Distractions

Chapter Fourteen

Weight Loss Schedules

Monkey Rituals

The Weight Loss Monkeys acknowledge that at various stages of life food can mean different things. For example, during childhood and adolescence, we tend to please our parents by finishing what is on our plates, even when we feel full.

Compared to other countries, in the United States food is abundant and often costs less than some of our other daily expenses. Under these conditions, food occasions are often used to celebrate meaningful events and provide excuses for us to unite with other people. Perhaps the most disturbing food reality is that celebrating or commiserating with food has become an uncontrollable practice.

A Self-portrait

My unhealthy food rituals were the result of random and unconscious negative emotions.

Overeating affected celebrations with my friends, during which I could intertwine both occasions: the celebration of the friendship and the depth of unresolved negative feelings. During these food occasions, I would be unfocused and select menu items that fit the event and not my diet plan.

Social Significance

Although wild monkeys are social creatures, they do not use food to be social; they use food strictly as a means of nourishment and survival. In contrast, many individuals use food beyond their survival instincts.

In urban areas, food consumption sometimes has little to do with relieving hunger and more to do with our need to endure our unhappy emotions. For example, eating sugary foods can be comforting, and drinking caffeine-laden beverages can produce a temporary spurt of energy. On the surface, these may appear to be reactions to our daily routines; however, I noticed that my cravings were prompted by a deep-rooted need to feel emotionally calm.

Corresponding with this, appearance also mattered, and I tended to choose those foods that both looked and tasted appetizing. The importance of food appearance can also be connected to events, during which certain distinct foods play recognizable roles. Examples of this include birthday cake versus sponge cake, or dining experiences in expensive restaurants, where the presentation of the food marks the occasion.

Celebrations also have social origins and are used primarily to cultivate relationships with other people. As is common practice, when I was younger my parents relied on food celebrations to entertain their friends. We usually served an array of decadent foods, which we never ate when we dined as a family. These foods were considered special, purchased to impress or create a more festive mood.

Food consciousness can also have strong associations with culture, location, and gender. I have noticed that as a female I tend to arrange and participate in more food gatherings. Being Indian, I cook customary ethnic foods. Using these examples, it became clear that I had more connections with food than just simple nutrition.

The Weight Loss Monkeys don't see anything wrong with socializing or congregating; they do this all the time. What they don't understand is why individuals must use food to have social experiences. Although the practice of celebrating with food may have a purpose, at some point in our history a change of routine and gathering practices resulted in food celebrations becoming essential to our interactions with other people.

It could be inferred that in our human world, the tendency to cultivate culinary experiences becomes significant to creating distractions and avoiding isolation.

Clock Celebrations

We no longer eat based on hunger. Our common food routines are a celebration of time.

There are very few meals I can remember eating because I was genuinely hungry or feeling low in energy. Here, the question to be asked is, why do we still eat when the body isn't asking for food?

Clock celebrations also impact diet effectiveness. Dieters who lead highly social lives are better served by planning meals and closely monitoring when they eat.

Time has produced common food events such as breakfast, lunch, and dinner. Let's not forget to mention snack times, which have become a significant component of certain diet plans, particularly those diets that require eating prepared meals.

These diets may not be suitable for highly social dieters, who may eat more food based on events rather than the time of day. In such situations, planning meals in advance becomes critical to diet success, particularly if the dieter travels for his or her work and must rely on the foods that are available at the travel destination.

Monkey Planning

Within our social patterns, dining out is often unavoidable. In these situations, diet management relies on greater awareness and our ability to make the best menu selections during special food circumstances.

Food planning before any social event can reduce the tendency to make unhealthy food choices that will potentially take the dieter out of health focus.

Another suggestion is to limit choices by ordering the same foods. An example of this is to decide which meals to eat in advance of the event—for example, choosing only salads at restaurants or eating from the raw vegetable platter at parties—and never deviating from this plan.

In most weight loss situations, planned eating can be viewed as a tool that helps to promote consistent and uninterrupted diet focus.

~ ~ ~

Identifying Unexpected Food Events

By using the Monkey tools, I became aware of how I continued to eat even when I was full.

I also noticed that I ate larger portions when I dined in restaurants because I had never paid attention to portion size.

Offering some background, an article produced by the CDC states that portion sizes began increasing in the 1970s "and have continued to do so." According to another article produced by Health and Age, plate sizes have also expanded; the average dinner plate has increased from seven to nine inches to eleven to twelve inches.[4]

Reinventing Time

Eating food because of time rituals is typically a human condition.

After I moved to America, I encountered the unique mealtime commonly referred to as brunch. This meal does not exist in other countries (not yet at least). The idea of combining breakfast and lunch with a smorgasbord of foods also supports the unconscious belief that missing a meal (breakfast) allows for eating more food at the next mealtime to make up for what we have missed.

Other common clock rituals include eating meals at certain times of the day—lunch around noon and dinner in the evening hours, usually after 6:00 p.m. Mealtimes also help to regulate food intake; however, they may also be responsible for our inability to experience actual hunger.

Alternative Diet Practices

Eating in a different way, even being on a specific food program (a regulated diet), is usually contrary to mainstream eating.

Becoming vegetarian or vegan or even following any diet plan is not considered mainstream and can often be perceived as socially awkward, particularly during celebration events with food.

As far as congregating is concerned, starting a new diet or health practice can sometimes feel uncomfortable. In addition, the dieter's efforts can also be undervalued by the people he or she chooses to dine with.

Although diet regimens are supportive of good health, they are difficult to incorporate as part of mainstream eating without having exceptional focus.

When I was dieting, the diets I chose were those that I could maintain in social settings. Of course, these plans were never successful because I learned nothing about food nutrition, particularly when I was eating the same foods as mainstream eaters.

Monkey Chapter Summary

Before starting any diet, review the food choices and create several food contingency plans. This includes deciding on alternate menu choices and stocking your pantry with the foods that are part of your chosen diet. These contingency plans reduce the impulse to eat decadent foods and keep the dieter focused on his or her health initiative.

Food preplanning also becomes essential for those dieters who often dine out or participate in social eating events.

The most valuable Monkey diet is always personalized and includes high-quality foods that are readily available.

The dieter's efforts to implement his or her diet may be undervalued by mainstream eaters and therefore requires exceptional focus to maintain and continue.

Eating based on clock time versus actual hunger delays the digestion process and ensures that the body must manage and dispose of more food than what it actually needs.

~ ~ ~

Monkey Chapter Notes

Chapter Fifteen

Out of Focus

Monkey Nostalgia

While on vacation and the heaviest I have ever been in my entire life, I became inspired to write this book and to use it to motivate myself to lose weight.

I knew that most commercial diet plans could yield results. What was disturbing was that throughout all of those years of dieting I had never been able to sustain my weight loss. This had nothing to do with the diet programs but more to do with my unwillingness to follow the diet instructions.

It had been my thoughts, in conjunction with my food behaviors, that had kept me emotionally unhappy and overweight.

There was no one to blame but myself for eating all of those extra portions, those many cupcakes or that millionth slice of bread loaded with butter. I had tasted these foods before, so why on earth was I eating them again?

Finally, I could not blame the diets for using food to be social or to compensate for my emotional highs and lows. I came to realize that the diets had not failed me—I had failed the diets!

The introduction to this book describes how establishing that connection between food and emotion changed my life. Having this knowledge improved my overall health focus, which resulted in better food behaviors. I learned that other people focused on nutrition and not diets as the foundation for their health initiatives. The illustration I used in a previous chapter described my friend who avoided mainstream foods and stayed fit, healthy, and at her perfect size and weight. She never viewed her food choices as a temporary fix, but as a lifetime practice. Although she ate mostly fruits and vegetables, she also ate high-quality meals, which included controlled portions of decadent foods. One bite of anything decadent and my friend was satisfied with that particular food experience. A second portion of anything was out of the question, and she never dined late in the evening or went to bed with a full stomach.

In contrast, fruits and vegetables were never foods that interested me. I had never taught myself to enjoy and respect them the way that she did.

I realized that it was a combination of these practices that kept healthy people not only slim but also fully food conscious. Cheating or overindulging were unheard-of concepts, and improved health was the outcome of being focused on a greater survival awareness.

Of course, mastering these lessons didn't happen overnight. Taste experiences had always been a huge part of my life, and this would not change if I continued to be social.

Focus and Awareness

When I started to live the life of focused health, I asked myself at what point food had become a distraction from my emotions. Perhaps the best answer here is that food was the only part of my life that I could rely on. Food was accessible, affordable, and in plentiful supply. I also didn't have to make an appointment with a therapist to deal with my emotional issues; I could just eat a chocolate bar or any other special food and my problems would go away, at least for that moment.

Weight gain had been the consistent and most unproductive outcome of overeating. Gaining weight was the final result, the equivalent of a coat of armor that appeared as layers of fat protecting me from painful past emotions.

The irony here was that without identifying these emotions and food patterns, I would never have been able to experience better health.

To Think Is to Be Human

The Weight Loss Monkeys don't have food and emotion connectors. They eat highly nutritious foods as a means to survive. Using an elevated sense of awareness, they view health as a natural consequence of being in harmony with this planet.

When I finally embraced the notion of health awareness, every aspect of my life changed. My weight loss improved, and I used the tools in this book to produce a greater diet focus. More important, my food selections now complemented my health initiative.

Does this cause me to avoid decadent foods? The answer is no.

Am I more conscious when I am exposed to decadent foods? The answer is most definitely yes!

What Are You Focused On?

Wild monkeys are always focused on survival.

They have natural instincts that discourage eating unhealthy foods. They inherently understand that if they eat the wrong foods their survival rate will diminish.

Monkey Perspective

In our typical Western food society, weight gain is 90 percent about our emotional health and 10 percent about food-related issues. Weight gain happens when there is an absence of a natural instinct to survive.

Monkey Questions: Focus

- List five reasons why you want to lose weight and rank these reasons by their levels of importance, number one being the most important reason.

a. ______________________________

b. ______________________________

c. ______________________________

d. ______________________________

e. ______________________________

- Have you ever been on a diet? Yes ( ) No ( )
- Do you want to lose weight? Yes ( ) No ( )

Write a detailed response to the following questions.

- Why do you want to lose weight?
- How many diets have you been on in your life? List the names of each of these diets.
- If diets equal desperation, and most diets work, what did not work when you were on a diet?
- Who are you losing weight for? Why do you believe these individuals are important to your physical health?

Monkey Action

- List five ways in which your life changes when you weigh less.

1. ____________________
2. ____________________
3. ____________________
4. ____________________
5. ____________________

- Post these five success answers in a place where you can review them every day.

Monkey Field Trip

Visit your local bookstore and count the number of diet books in the health section. Write this number down in your thoughts log, as well as your reaction to this number.

Have you maintained all of the weight that you have lost in the past?

Has the availability of so many diets helped your weight loss in the past? If so, how?

Diet-stops

A dieter's distractions can result in a lack of commitment to the chosen diet plan. The Weight Loss Monkeys call this the diet-stop.

From a marketing perspective, if dieters completely stop their diets, they can always begin a different plan. This belief is what has kept the weight loss industry creative and accessible.

For decades, I had been a yo-yo dieter. I cheated and failed many diets. The need to start a new diet or food fad diminished when I became focused on nutrition. I then understood the importance of having a survival instinct, which in turn caused me to eliminate many of those special foods that had interrupted my weight loss in the past.

What Is Your Plan?

The diet plan is merely the tool. When used as designed, this tool can produce improved health conditions. This is considered a lifetime plan, which should be simple to use, offer palatable foods to eat, and can be customized to accommodate boredom and lifestyle changes.

Continuing this plan will depend on access to regular exercise and to those foods that are required by the plan. This new plan also incorporates motivational tools during various stages of weight loss. Being motivated reduces the impact of "special" food temptations, unplanned eating events, and the problems faced after reaching weight loss plateaus.

What You Will Need

The Weight Loss Monkeys urge you to buy a good quality weight scale, to weigh yourself every day, and to record these results on your weight loss tracking tool.

What You Will Not Need

The chosen diet or health plan should not rely on special supplements, surgeries, or ingesting foods produced using antibiotics or hormones.

A New Diet World

Maintaining a new diet may not be easy. Keep in mind, wild monkeys have had the same eating plan for generations, and they are not about to change it in a moment. When I began my health initiative, the adjustment from social eating to a plan that focused on eating for good health required focus and practice. To improve results, I was required to make modifications to both the foods I ate and my exercise routine.

I became inspired to lose weight after I identified my Monkey factor, the core reason for my overeating behaviors.

Building a health focus also helped to identify my undirected wants, and with them, my tendency to gravitate toward fad diets. I began a health initiative to discourage these tendencies, which then resulted in beginning slow and steady weight loss—a concept that I had never embraced in the past.

Finding exercises that I enjoyed required research and practice. Finally, fitting into smaller clothes sizes took months to achieve.

The most challenging aspect of this new health initiative was adjusting my taste buds to eat foods that were viewed as nutritious versus "special."

Emotional Focus

Without identification, undirected wants will always deplete diet concentration. When I ate foods that were not on my chosen food plan, I wrote about these events and corresponding emotions in my thoughts log. This information allowed me to become more alert and to gradually avoid repeat incidents of overeating.

Because certain food experiences were often rooted in emotional events, it could take several eating cycles to identify each unproductive food memory.

To provide a few general examples, cheesecake may have an emotional link to a happy memory with your grandma. Eating a hamburger on a sunny Fourth of July or other similar food experiences create nostalgic taste emotions. The memory could be so far in our past that it may take repeating these events to properly identify them. However, after isolating these exposed food triggers, I was encouraged to implement healthier food behaviors that could counteract any tendency to overeat.

Too Much to Eat

Social events often result in random exposure to decadent foods. In my situation, I realized that social events with food would not change, so I had to. I needed to improve my food awareness and to take responsibility for those emotional highs and lows that triggered my overeating.

Selecting a salad by choice versus eating a cupcake in reaction to a food trigger signals a heightened awareness. The same situation applies to when we choose fresh fruit or sorbet instead of a slice of cheesecake.

When new food behaviors became established, my undirected wants had less influence. From this point forward, the awareness of any new food response represented a powerful shift in my eating consciousness.

Monkey Questions: Discussion

These questions have been repeated from other chapters in this book because the responses will change as the dieter's health focus improves.

Try to write detailed answers to these two questions.

- Do you really want to lose weight and why?
- How much weight do you want to lose and for whom?

Monkey Chapter Summary

When survival consciousness is diminished, this results in both living and eating out of focus.

Permanent weight loss often relies on identifying emotional eating.

The identification process supports the success of any new diet program.

Having negative food thoughts is the main reason why dieters continue to eat "special," decadent foods, and succumb to bouts of overeating.

Weight loss focus takes time to acquire because connecting food memories to taste requires diligent practice. Food focus produces the awareness that will eventually lead to healthier food behaviors.

~ ~ ~

Monkey Chapter Notes

Chapter Sixteen

Monkey Say No More

Monkey Dialogue

The results on the scale (good or bad) always promote dialogue.

The Say Monkey encourages food conversations with food mentors and alternative eaters to gain support and encouragement during the diet process and beyond.

I have heard people discuss their weight loss successes with enthusiasm, which has caused me to feel discouraged about my own results. This changed when I became aware of my food thoughts and subsequent emotional reactions. In this new healthy thought environment, I was able to harness my focus by increasing my diet motivation.

Positive food dialogue includes discussions about both weight loss and weight gain. Because other people's reactions cannot be anticipated, it becomes difficult to determine just how these reactions will impact the dieter's weight loss focus. In these situations, adding motivational tools maintains diet consistency by creating a greater health focus.

How Monkey Dialogue Works

Example 1: "I have gained a pound" or "I have lost a pound."

As it pertains to the final goal weight, this form of dialogue is not significant. To improve focus, I introduced Monkey markers to guide my conversations with other people.

Example 2: "I have lost ten pounds" or "I am one size smaller than I was three months ago."

Monkey Discussion

1. For one week avoid discussing your weight with anyone.

2. If you must discuss either your diet or health initiative, write down (in the margins or at the back of this book) why this subject came up and who you talked to. Identify why you feel the need to discuss your weight with certain people and what role these people represent in your life.

3. If you discuss weight loss and weight gain, what feelings and emotions surface? Examples include frustration, insecurity, embarrassment, or feelings of isolation.

Monkey Chapter Summary

Individuals who maintain their ideal weight rarely discuss their weight issues with other people.

The Say Monkey discourages random conversations about diet progress. This will help to strengthen the dieter's food focus.

Diet dialogue is encouraged with food mentors and alternative eaters to improve knowledge and motivation.

Writing in the Monkey thoughts log identifies food emotion triggers that may cause diet distractions.

~ ~ ~

Chapter Seventeen

Is Your Body Talking to You?

A Self-portrait

I didn't realize that my body was talking to me until I reached my early forties.

At that time, I was the heaviest weight I had ever been, and during that weight-gain period, my body's aches and pains were at their greatest.

Being overweight made it difficult to participate in exercise. My feet tired easily, and many mornings my legs hurt when I got out of bed. Even though I felt energetic, over time my physical limitations became more acute.

Because I had also grown two clothes sizes in eighteen months, the list of physical complaints continued to increase. The most noticeable of these complaints was a deterioration of my natural body systems, which resulted in uncomfortable and sometimes embarrassing situations. My digestion slowed, and gas and bloating became as frequent as every day. My stomach sometimes hurt after eating meat or heavy dairy foods, and I also developed an acid-reflux-type condition. The most surprising discovery was that I couldn't drink large amounts of water without having a bathroom close by.

Monkey Migration

Another unusual side effect was that the foods that I loved no longer tasted the same. This wasn't because my taste buds had changed but because there was something wrong with the taste of certain food ingredients. Cakes tasted fatty rather than spongy, and chicken took longer to chew. Not only were the foods not tasty, but my body was not adapting to them.

A large majority of the foods in our common Western diet are not structurally the same foods that we ate a decade ago. To offer a distinct contrast, monkeys living in the wild still eat the same foods their ancestors ate. In this natural habitat, the food sources have never changed. What has changed is food availability, as their habitat shrinks in size and is replaced with urban areas.

As it relates to food quality, it is more likely that the wild monkey population will become extinct due to starvation rather than physical disorders or diseases.

The reason why people living in urban areas are no longer eating foods their forefathers ate is because a large majority of these foods are now processed or produced using chemicals.

In our new millennium, food quality is the poorest it has ever been, and the Weight Loss Monkeys believe there exists a noticeable relationship between food quality and modern disease.

Food First Aid

Wild monkeys do not eat foods that have unnatural ingredients. In contrast, people living in urban areas eat foods that they cannot even identify, pronounce, spell, or digest properly. Inspecting certain food labels reveals ingredient names that do not even resemble common foods.

Those of us who consume processed and chemically laden foods suffer the consequences. Constipation, water retention, acid reflux, and any other number of food-related issues compromise our health and impede the efficiency of our metabolism.

To improve our bodies' functionality, the Weight Loss Monkeys believe health risks can be reduced if we eat foods that are naturally produced. There are no absolutes when it comes to perfect food consumption. The suggested Monkey rule is to eat fewer processed foods and to strictly avoid consuming those foods that are produced with pesticides and bulking agents.

Monkey Chapter Summary

It is unknown what the combined reactions are when we consume chemicals that are connected to the fertilizers and pesticides that are used to create our food supply. Under these conditions, the simpler the foods consumed, the better! If the natural world didn't create the food naturally, then it follows that people, who are part of the natural world, are not meant to eat these unnatural foods.

~ ~ ~

Monkey Chapter Notes

Monkey Do

Chapter Eighteen

Monkey Action

"Acceptance means: For now, this is what this situation, this moment requires me to do, and so I do it willingly."

—Eckhart Tolle

Monkey Do Does It the Best!

The Do Monkey does whatever is necessary to maintain diet focus. This focus increases when there is motivation.

Diet motivation can also be described as creative thinking, which inspires action. Increasing diet creativity allows us to make changes to our food programs so that we can achieve weight loss and reach our health goals.

During the diet process, there may be times when our focus might be better or worse, but the doing is what ultimately allows us to continue on the plan.

Getting weighed is part of that plan and provides a measurement of both success and failure. Not enough weight lost over a long period of time may require reviewing the overall weight management process and making modifications.

Although the effects of metabolism, age, and hormones play a significant role in weight gain and slowing weight loss, the basic nature of weight management remains elemental. The conventional theory is that a reduction of consumed calories with added exercise will eventually result in weight loss.

Many of us want to lose weight, but eating less than what our mind instructs us to eat may be the greatest challenge. We eat more food because we believe we need more food, not to survive but to manage our emotions and interact with others.

Do Monkey Tips

1. Eat foods that promote healthy weight loss. Prepare these foods so they are visually appealing and palatable. This, as well as food variety, will ensure that you stay on track while on the diet.
2. Motivation helps to improve thought clarity, and this will encourage the use of other diet tools such as exercise, better recipes, and menu planning.
3. If you enjoy sugary sweets, the diet you choose should replace the usual sugary foods with healthy, satisfying alternatives.
4. Make foods look appetizing so that you avoid food boredom. Dress up desserts, or do what is necessary to make these foods look and taste good. This rule also applies to savory, salty, fatty, and fried foods, which you may need to replace with satisfying alternatives.

5. Weigh, weigh, weigh everything, this includes you! Buy good quality and accurate scales.
6. Fix snacks that you love and that meet the goals of your diet or health initiative. Try to stay full and satisfied so that you don't eat the wrong foods.
7. The impact of undirected wants may cause the dieter to eat quickly. Chewing helps but requires patience and practice. Start with a minimum of ten chews per mouthful, building up to twenty-five or more.
8. Stay full. Drink plenty of water. People on diets tend to get hungry faster. This may have something to do with the influence of taste. Feeling full can be challenging when we believe that certain foods are unpalatable or when they are presented to us in smaller portions. Monkey fill food includes salad and drinking water as part of the meal experience.

Monkey Questions: Diet Creativity

Write detailed answers to these questions.

- Why and when do your food cravings happen? Record these dates and the events in your thoughts log.
- Are you a food participant or a bystander? Participants plan for food events in advance; the bystander is unprepared and allows food events to just happen, which results in overeating.
- What do you eat during these food events?

Do you enjoy sweet, sour, salty, or fatty foods? Do you eat more of one particular food type? Which type, and how often?

- How many times in any month do these food events occur? Are you responsible for initiating these food events, and if so, why?
- Do these eating events involve people, and who are they?
- Some people eat more when they are alone. Are you one of them?
- If you usually eat alone, do you need to add more social activities to your life so you avoid eating out of boredom or loneliness?
- Are there Do activities that may motivate and encourage you not to overeat? List the Do activities that interest you.

Monkey Chapter Summary

The Do Monkey tools encourage continuous motivation as a way to maintain diet focus. It is more difficult to arrive at a remote destination if we do not have a map and working compass. The Do Monkey tools represent the motivation map and compass used during the dieter's weight loss journey.

~ ~ ~

Monkey Chapter Notes

Chapter Nineteen

Monkey Movement

Building Momentum

During my twenties, benefiting from regular exercise meant attending classes organized by my favorite aerobic instructor. This particular instructor could be described as big, burly, and Samoan. Most important, he was an oh-so-cool dude. The very the moment he walked into any room the air literally buzzed with excitement.

During his classes, this instructor opted to use energetic and recognizable music, which bolstered his popularity. This music included a mixture of funk and pop, which at the time was the best music to exercise to. The beat alone would ensure excessive synchronized bopping about, which resulted in an excellent workout.

Most of these classes ran for more than an hour, and I experienced all of those exercise-related benefits. I sweated; my muscles ached beautifully; and I did a lot of heavy breathing, checking my heart rate whenever the instructor insisted.

The most important benefit was that I went to as many of this instructor's classes as I could pack into my schedule and was happy to stay until the very end. I never became bored, and I was proud to consider myself one of his groupies.

This instructor's success had everything to do with his ability to inspire and motivate. Needless to say, his classes were both encouraging and supportive to my weight loss, which also allowed me to maintain my health goals.

Historically, I have never been a fan of anything athletic. My first excuse is that I was raised in the seventies, in a country and a time when exercise was not considered important or essential to longevity. In contrast, in California, where I live now, daily exercise is considered as important as brushing the teeth.

The true test became time. At age thirteen, I remember taking a judo class that was a gruesome one hour of tussling about on a mat. However, aerobics with an inspired instructor made getting hot and sweaty much more fun. This comparison has nothing to do with the art of judo but with my level of enjoyment of certain forms of exercise.

In my thirties, my views on exercise became part of managing my health, and it was then that I discovered that exercise was essential to losing weight.

When I became aware of this, it felt like I had been handed a miracle cure. In hindsight, what I had been handed was another very valuable tool, which I needed to use regularly in order to experience a lasting effect.

As an added bonus, I realized that with daily exercise my body image would also improve.

Of course, without exercise it would become more and more difficult to maintain firm muscle mass, which would result in fat accumulating in very undesirable areas of my body.

Most significant, I noticed that when I didn't exercise my food diet worked less efficiently, and my weight loss slowed.

Monkey Movement

Unlike the regularity of mealtimes (customarily three times a day), I never viewed exercise as a daily must-do practice.

At some point, my thoughts had fixed on the idea that I needed food more than I needed exercise to survive. To make matters worse, I had always viewed exercise as an event that had to be planned, like going to the movies on a Friday night. Because of these old thoughts, food and exercise were never presented as two complementary components that when combined resulted in improved health.

The Monkey thoughts log, used in conjunction with my customized health initiative, produced those creative ideas that allowed me to explore new kinds of physical movements that I could both enjoy and maintain.

Since food was available and plentiful, physical exertion required much more focus, particularly when I had never considered this important to my overall health.

The weight loss tracking tool provided a visual mechanism that identified how much slower my weight loss became when I didn't exercise. These numbers also identified when I consumed more calories than I expended in energy. At various times during my diet, I was eating too much for my activity level and as a result not losing weight.

In contrast, wild monkeys rely on activities that are complementary to their survival instincts and specific to their environments. They store very little of the food they digest because they use most of it for energy. Following the wild monkey rule, exercise should never be viewed as a maybe activity.

Our Physical Limits

Wild monkeys use most of their bodies to exert physical momentum, and the human physique is equally flexible. There are many forms of enjoyable exercise that can produce an improved health focus and at the same time expend enough energy to promote weight loss.

Using these guidelines, the first question to ask is: Which exercises to choose? The second is: Which of these exercises will support continuous good health?

Exercise Choices

The choice of exercise is limited by personal health factors, as well as the time available to complete the exercise routine. Under these conditions, choosing just the right exercise may not happen in an instant and may require investigation and practice.

Monkey Questions: Exercise

Instructions: Write concise answers to each question. Do not overwrite. Be specific and honest.

- Why do you think exercise will be helpful in reaching your health goal?
- What types of exercise have you done in the past that you enjoy?
- Do you consider yourself physically heavy or light?

Why do you believe this? Did you learn this somewhere, or is this true?

- Are you too heavy to start certain exercise programs, and if so, which ones?
- List the exercise programs that you enjoy and that you can physically accomplish?
- Which of these exercises can you start immediately?
- What exercise does your doctor recommend?
- Are the exercises you have chosen supportive to your weight loss goal?
- How much time can you reasonably devote to exercise? Be specific and honest.

Monkey Tasks

- Create a personal exercise schedule. This can be modified as needed.
- Exercising takes time. Explain how you will make adjustments to your daily routine so that exercise becomes an important, must-do activity?

- During the weight loss process, when do you think you will be able to safely increase exercising so that you can improve your health results? Write down the date when this change is scheduled to happen.

Monkey Exercise Affirmation

I always choose exercises that are safe, realistic, and fit into my schedule.

Monkey Chapter Summary

Physical mobility is essential to improving our survival instinct. The exercise style chosen must be safe, physically supportive to continuous weight loss, and result in reaching the overall health goal.

Exercise must be enjoyable and sustainable.

Exercise can be modified to support weight loss progress.

Exercise is both a planned-for and must-do activity.

Monkey Note

Your health and safety are the number-one priority. The Weight Loss Monkeys and I are not doctors, therapists, physiologists, or scientists. Please seek the advice of a professional before beginning any new diet or exercise program. We do not advocate starting any exercise program that is unduly strenuous. Although this may be tempting to do, this may also result in injury and initiate undirected wants that interrupt weight loss focus.

~ ~ ~

Always check with your doctor
before starting any new exercise, diet or health plan!

~ ~ ~

Monkey Chapter Notes

Monkey Movement

Chapter Twenty

Organization & Routines

A Self-portrait

The moment I began any diet, I wanted it to be over. Most of all, I wanted all of those extra pounds to be gone without making any sacrifices.

After weeks of "focused" dieting, the results were not always promising. I wished the number on the scale was smaller; I felt dismal because I didn't fit into smaller clothes sizes; and most important, I was never satisfied with my weight loss results.

There were times when my friends lost weight and I would offer them encouragement. Secretly, I would envy them for making all of those sacrifices, shedding the pounds, and looking thinner. My mind would become overwhelmed with unhelpful thoughts. How could it be okay for them to get healthy and thin while I was stuck at the same weight? Why was I giving them encouragement, but when I lost one or two pounds it was never enough?

Usually it was not until I was already overweight that I started a new diet. I had been at this place before and it always felt the same, cycles of overeating followed by cycles of extreme deprivation.

Monkey Perspective

The Weight Loss Monkeys believe that unrealistic weight loss expectations are the beginning of the end. How people gain weight and lose weight is based on a variety of factors, the least important of which is how much we deprive our bodies of the decadent foods that we love.

Accelerated diets that guarantee drastic weight loss often do not offer guidelines for food discipline and weight maintenance. Also, many of the more familiar commercial plans that offer miracle shakes and diet supplements promote quick fixes rather than a permanent lifestyle change.

A Dieter's Results

During all of my diet experiences, quick-fix diets produced only rapid weight loss and a boost to my ego. After I lost the initial five to ten pounds, my expectations were often greater than the actual weight lost. More often than not, the rest of the weight would come off more slowly, and the goal always seemed harder to achieve. Under these conditions, the numbers that registered on the scale could never be fully appreciated.

Monkey Weight

The Weight Loss Monkeys are naturally fit and never overweight, underweight, impoverished, or disease-ridden. Their ideal weight represents a way of life.

Their consciousness is never focused on food, so their health goals correspond to a heightened survival instinct.

Focus Versus Emotion

People tend to eat more because they have a wide spectrum of thoughts that are based on emotions. In contrast, monkeys living in the wild are primitive and do not have the mental capabilities to experience excessive emotion. To compensate for not having complex emotions they have heightened instincts, and this is why they tend not to overeat.

When it comes to being on a diet, controlling excessive emotions becomes essential to improving weight loss.

The more weight lost, the more motivation needed. When there exists a positive thought environment, negative emotions become less influential and awareness increases.

Time Beyond the Clock

Significant and lasting weight loss relies on time management. As this applies to weight loss and health, more time is needed to incorporate new diet foods and other diet-related behaviors such as exercise. Adding a time component improves diet focus and discourages unrealistic expectations.

Without improved time management, permanent weight loss will always be difficult to manage.

Productive Diet Time = Weight Loss Success

Scheduling Your Diet

Before choosing the final nutrition plan, I needed to make sure that I had enough time to manage the entire health initiative, which included exercise and motivational practices.

I had to revisit all of my diet routines, particularly how, when, and why I ate food.

Time Management = Managed Weight Loss

Monkey Time Management Tool

The following is a general list of time issues to consider when starting a new weight loss plan.

- Enough food preparation time (for buying and preparing foods).
- Correct and regular exercise for weight loss (a must).
- Sleep. Significant sleep is critical to overall health and the efficiency of your metabolism.
- Rest (not the same as sleep). Getting adequate amounts of rest improves focus. At least two five-minute rest periods every day. Rest equals Monkey stillness (Chapter Eleven).
- An abundant amount of emotional support. This includes scheduling time with positive people who will support your weight loss efforts.
- Sufficient diet finances (to purchase healthier foods, exercise equipment, gym and club memberships, etc.).
- Daily motivation. Time for affirmations and meditation, which helps to improve diet focus.

- Daily weigh-ins (this should be at the same time every day). Daily weigh-ins help to monitor water retention and unusual food sensitivities that interrupt weight loss.

Monkey Weight Loss Schedule

The best way to create enough time for any diet program is to ensure that the chosen health plan complements your existing routines.

The new diet or health initiative must be adjusted for life and family commitments. The Food Time Management Tool (Figure. 4.) can assist the dieter with event scheduling and improve awareness of food responses during specific situations.

Monkey Routine

Diet time management flows naturally after the new weight loss diet behaviors have been established. However, these routines may require modification when weight loss becomes impacted by metabolic adjustments or when there are weight loss interruptions. More time adjustment may also be required at the later stages of your program when increasing exercise may be necessary to improving weight loss results.

Staying on Track

The Monkey tools can help the dieter stay on the diet and improve his or her awareness of time management.

Most of the Monkey Say and Do tools are designed as thought stabilizers. The most popular stabilizing tools include meditation, affirmations, goal awareness, mantras, prayer, exercise, therapy, food mentors, and other forms of positive motivation.

Improving Focus

During weight loss, my routines were supported by the tracking process and those other tools that I had committed to.

Using these tools allowed me to focus less on the destination and more on the journey.

The goal remained always in sight (taped onto my scale and my computer).

I knew that losing twenty pounds in one month was unrealistic based on such factors as age, level of activity, and the efficiency of my body.

Everyday use of the Weight Loss Tracking Tool (Chapter 7) identified how much weight my body could lose in a specific period of time.

Finally, after using the affirmations and meditation tools, it became less likely to harbor false expectations that might take me out of diet focus.

Monkey Thresholds

The Weight Loss Monkeys consider slow weight loss the most reliable. Slow weight loss allows the body's metabolism to adjust to new thresholds that are sometimes called plateaus.

Diet plateaus as positive indicators. Reaching a plateau is a time for celebration because the plateau indicates that the dieter must make adjustments to his or her food and exercise plans.

Weight Loss Plateau + Time = Continued Diet Success + Celebration!

Monkey Task

Create your diet schedule by including the day-to-day conditions that may impact your diet. Be honest and specific. Do not agree to diet activities that may be difficult for you to achieve. Use the Monkey time management tool as a rough outline of your schedule. Make adjustments whenever necessary.

Monkey Chapter Summary

The diet is the first thing that will be sacrificed when life routines, emotional upsets, and social events impact the dieter's time schedule.

Having a weight loss management plan becomes critical to consistent weight loss. This plan should be flexible and easy to adjust, particularly when there are weight loss plateaus.

~ ~ ~

Food Time Management Tool

Week Ending ______________________________

Date (1)	Event Type (2)	Time Scale (hrs) (3)	Food Required (yes or no) (4)	Other Factors (5)	Bystander (B) Participant (P) (6)

Fig. 4. Food Time Management Tool (Make Copies)

Food Time Management Tool Instructions

1. Date: Weekly schedule.
2. Event Type: Examples include parties, eating-out events (breakfasts, brunches, lunches, and dinners), and business meetings.
3. Time Scale: Event times in hours. For full-day events or vacations, use multiple sheets for preplanning.
4. Food required: Will you need to preplan your food needs for each event?
5. Other Factors: Conditions that prevent food planning. How will you cope with food during these events?
6. Bystander or Participant: To be completed after the event. This column tracks your food-planning progress.

Monkey Chapter Notes

Chapter Twenty-one

The Choosy Monkey

Because I Can Right Now!

It didn't take long for me to realize that I could do whatever I wanted when it came to food. Even if I'd tasted cheesecake a hundred times, I could have it again, and again and again.

With or without full awareness, we make our own choices. The selection process can be so random that many of the foods we pick are not even part of our diets. These choices can be endless and varied, from a cupcake to a slice of cheesecake, a brownie to a cinnamon roll, even healthy choices like soup or salad with a sandwich. At the movies, we can pick the small, medium, or large (even extra large) soda and/or popcorn. At Thanksgiving dinner (my favorite), we often get to pick between dark or white turkey meat. We also get to pick quantities, one cupcake or two, and let's not forget the vast selections of ice cream.

This realization prompted a visit to the local grocery store. I was shocked to count over fifty varieties of bread. Some of the breads were identical, but they were made and packaged by different companies.

There appears to be no end to our fascination with food. Offering one last example, consider that we can roast, boil, bake, or poach a chicken. We not only get to choose chicken, but we get to decide exactly how it will be cooked. When it comes to food, unless we live in a starving society, choice at this moment is not an issue. If anything, choice is part of our obesity problem, and it is also part of the solution.

Diet Confusion

Even when it came to the actual diets, I was always overwhelmed by all the choices. There were pill diets, shake diets, protein diets, and all-veggie diets. There were also programs that touted weight loss testimonials and clinically tested breakthroughs.

Given all of these choices, I could do whatever I wanted when it came to how I selected a new diet program. I could even switch programs if I became unhappy with my weight loss progress.

What made the situation more confusing was that all of these programs contradicted one another. Although they addressed opposing views on how to manage food, they hardly ever approached the subjects of how to maintain weight loss or deal with future body-shape issues.

A New Response

It would appear that the complement to having choice is not having choice. In other countries around the world, people do not have as many food varieties as we do. Even wild animals such as monkeys only have four or five categories of food. Their nutritional needs are met by eating a majority of fruits and green, leafy vegetables.

Knowing this, why couldn't I just wait and have ice cream after I had reached and maintained my goal weight? With so many varieties and flavors to chose from, there was little chance of ice cream becoming extinct! Also, why not stop thinking about certain foods altogether? Of course, this would be challenging, but the only sensible way to resist unhealthy foods would be to accept that I could eat them later if I wanted.

It was also true that I could have many flavors of ice cream, but I realized that I just didn't have to have ice cream at that moment. After I understood this, ignoring my food triggers became easier, because I knew that when it came to food, I could do whatever I wanted, whenever I wanted.

Monkey Identity

Wild monkeys always live in the present moment. Eckhart Tolle describes this present moment as "The Now." They live this way because they are primitive, and having a heightened sense of survival dictates that they must live with the resources at their disposal.

As far as weight loss is concerned, they have no fixed memories about what body type they should have. They also recognize their fears by using keen instinct. In contrast, throughout my life, I had stored away my fears as thought testimonials linked to unhappy food emotions created in my past.

Monkeys, as primitive creatures, have fewer complex emotions, which allows them to better manage their priorities. The main issues that they contend with are eating, sleeping, and surviving, not necessarily in that order. They remain social and involved in their family groups, and on purpose do not socialize with other species of animals.

Monkeys couldn't care less about body image, the opinions of others, or the influence of outside forces. In contrast, people tend to absorb these issues in a sponge-like manner. They crave acceptance, appreciation, love, consideration, and collaboration, and extend their social boundaries in order to assimilate with other cultures and the corresponding cultural foods.

Not every food is good for us, allowed on our diets, or necessary for maintaining better health. Food consumption has become random and compulsive. An example of this would be eating Chinese food on Monday, pizza on Tuesday, and a hamburger with fries on Wednesday. Being part of a large cultural food community has created attachments to a greater variety of foods that are not otherwise available in societies where food sources are limited. These foods, combined with this type of varied eating also serve to distract us from the balanced nutritional needs of our bodies. Under these conditions, the health issues become more pronounced and risk of diet failure becomes more frequent.

Diet focus now relies not only on how much we eat, but also on which foods can satisfy our food triggers, and how we eat when we are influenced by excessive choice.

Monkey Chapter Summary

Taking responsibility for our weight loss is the first step to a permanent weight loss solution. It is at this juncture that food memories weaken their influence and the ability to choose healthy foods becomes part of an improved instinct to survive.

Choice and random food selection always impact diet focus. Food choice is therefore influenced by such factors as the exact moment of choice and our food expectations, regardless of where we happen to be during our weight loss journey.

~ ~ ~

Monkey Chapter Notes

Chapter Twenty-two

Important and Necessary

Many of life's weight loss issues gravitate toward the finite expression of whether something is important or necessary.

When it comes to weight loss, important versus necessary is an integral component to long-term success and social food interaction.

In my life, having an established diet focus became important to having positive long-term food behaviors. Eating the correct foods was also important to my overall health.

An important health focus became the foundation to helping me create a spectrum of new food behaviors. This perspective compensated for the negative influence of undirected wants, which in the past had caused me to fail my diets.

As an example of the important and necessary ideology, breathing is one of those distinctions that can assume both. For people and wild monkeys, if we are unable to breathe then we die.

In the end, the decision to win the weight loss game will be up to us. How many slices of cheesecake and pizza are truly important when it comes to reaching our health goal? After we have already tasted these foods hundreds of times, is it important or even necessary for us to eat them again? Surely it is both important and necessary to eat fruits and vegetables, but do we?

Important and necessary also requires focusing on avoiding unhealthy foods, which are better saved for special occasions and not eaten every day.

These ideas take hold after we begin to use support tools such as exercise, meditation, affirmations, and note-taking. When using these tools as part of a consistent practice, health awareness improves and we become better able to manage our weight and any future weight loss issues.

Is it important and necessary to make motivation a practice?

Without motivation, continuing on the plan and staying at the goal weight may become challenging.

Healthy relationships are also important and necessary. Unless we live in solitary confinement, interaction with others becomes an important contributor to our emotional stability. When it comes to the subject of food management, is it necessary to be in an unhealthy relationship or important to be in a healthy one? That said, does it become important and necessary (if not vital) to surround ourselves with food mentors and fewer mainstream eaters?

Monkey Finale

The ability to eat nutritious food and drink good quality water is important to sustaining long life and better health. It is well-known that eating certain important foods will help us to live longer. In contrast, soft drinks, pizza, and cheesecake are not important foods, nor are they necessary to maintaining a long life.

As a society that is living longer, many of us are dying from mysterious diseases that cannot be cured with even the most promising medicines. Under these conditions, picking the right foods could be viewed as transcending even important and necessary.

Monkeys and other animals that live in their natural habitats do not die of cancer, Alzheimer's disease, or any other number of modern human illnesses that diminish the mind and rot the body. The fruits and green, leafy vegetables they eat do not come labeled with nutritional content information or any hazardous warning signs. In contrast, for most of us living in urban areas, food continues to be in plentiful and accessible supply, and based on what we are eating, has become a risk to our health. It would seem both important and necessary for general food quality to arrive in its purest form simply to prevent chronic illness.

In the final outcome, nourishing our bodies is the most essential component of how we choose the foods we eat. Taking control of our health and managing nutrition become both important and necessary to how long and how productively we live our lives.

~ ~ ~

Also Available from Bright Performance:

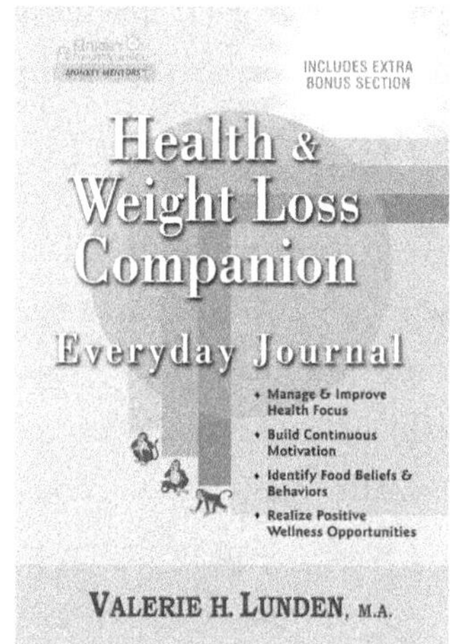

Health & Weight Loss Companion, Everyday Journal

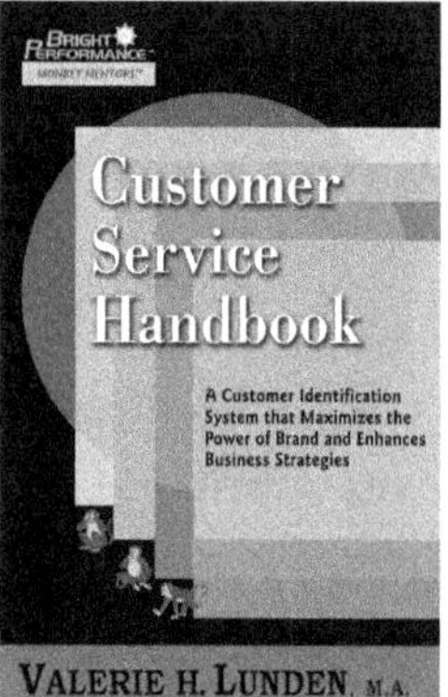

Consumer Service Handbook

To Purchase, visit BrightPerformance.com

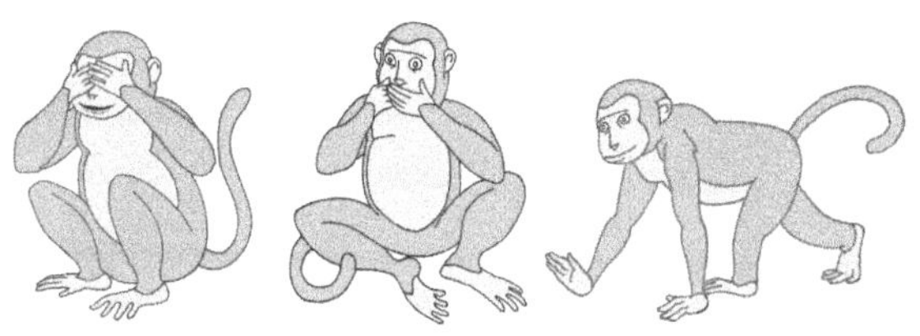

For workshop information, program support or other Monkey Mentor products, visit
www.brightperformance.com

Notes

Chapter One

1."Gene similarity." Frequently asked questions: Chimpanzee and Human Communication Institute, 2004. Accessible at: http://www.cwu.edu/cwuchci:faq.html.

Chapter Two

2. *Green for Life* by Victoria Boutenko.

Chapter Seven

3. Height and weight tables of the Metropolitan Life Insurance Company, 1983. From Western Bariatric. http://www.westernbariatricinstitute.com/default/Weight_Loss_Surgery_General/Weight_Loss_Surgery/Am_I_A_Candidate_For_Surgery/Height_Weight_Chart.

Chapter Fourteen

4. "Dinner plate expanding." Article produced by Health and Age. Accessible at: http://www.health-and-age.org/health-topics-/2006/2/10/dinner-plates-s.

Bibliography

Boutenko, Victoria. *Green for Life*. Oregon: Raw Family Publishing 2005.

Campbell, T. Colin, Ph.D. *The China Study*. Texas: Benbella Books 2004.

Cordain, Loren, Ph.D. *The Paleo Diet*. New Jersey: John Wiley & Sons, Inc. 2002.

Furhman, Joel, M.D. *Eat to Live*. New York: Little Brown and Company 2003.

Gott, Peter H, MD. *Dr Gott's No Flour No Sugar Diet*. New York: Hachette Books Group USA 2006.

Kristal, Harold, D.D.S, and James M. Haig, N.C. *The Nutrition Solution*. California: North Atlantic Books 2002.

Pollock, Dennis. *Overcoming Runaway Blood Sugar*. Oregon: Harvest House Publishers 2006.

Pratt, Steven, MD, and Kathy Mathews. *Super Foods*. New York: Harper Publishers 2005.

Tolle, Eckhart. *The Power of Now*. Canada: Namaste Publishing 2004.

Tolle, Eckhart. *A New Earth*. New York: Plume 2006.

Williams, Roger J., PhD. *Biochemical Individuality*. Texas: The University of Texas 1998.

Wolcott, William and Trish Fahey. *The Metabolic Typing Diet*. New York: Broadway Books 2000.

Young, Robert O., and Shelly Redford Young. *The pH Miracle*. New York: Warner Wellness 2002.

Monkey Chapter Notes

www.ingramcontent.com/pod-product-compliance
Lightning Source LLC
LaVergne TN
LVHW050630100826
845148LV00011B/1818

* 9 7 8 0 9 8 2 2 5 3 9 0 8 *